Chinese Medicine for Childhood Anxiety and Depression

CHINESE MEDICINE for CHILDHOOD ANXIETY and DEPRESSION

A PRACTICAL GUIDE FOR PRACTITIONERS AND PARENTS

REBECCA AVERN

Foreword by ELISA ROSSI

Illustrated by SARAH HOYLE

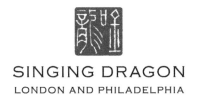

SINGING DRAGON

LONDON AND PHILADELPHIA

First published in Great Britain in 2022 by Singing Dragon,
an imprint of Jessica Kingsley Publishers
An Hachette Company

2

Disclaimer: The information contained in this book is not intended to replace the services of
trained medical professionals or to be a substitute for medical advice. The complementary therapy
described in this book may not be suitable for everyone to follow. You are advised to consult a
doctor before embarking on any complementary therapy programme and on any matters relating
to your health, and in particular on any matters that may require diagnosis or medical attention.

A CIP catalogue record for this title is available from the
British Library and the Library of Congress

ISBN 978 1 78775 781 3
eISBN 978 1 78775 782 0

Printed and bound by CPI Group (UK) Ltd, Croydon, CR0 4YY

Jessica Kingsley Publishers
Carmelite House
50 Victoria Embankment
London EC4Y 0DZ

www.singingdragon.com

In memory of my mother, who passed away while I was writing this book.

And to my father – from whom I have been physically separated due to COVID-19 and emotionally separated due to Alzheimer's.

I miss you both.

Contents

Foreword

Chinese medicine's wisdom can have an enormously positive impact on children's mental and emotional health.

Rebecca Avern unfolds this knowledge in *Chinese Medicine for Childhood Anxiety and Depression*, a book that has given me real pleasure, to my mind and to my heart.

Rebecca cares for children, parents and practitioners. She knows that we are all struggling, and that we do it in different ways. So, as practitioners or parents, we have to look at the individual baby, child or teenager; 'labels' are of no use. We are first invited to listen, observe, be curious, and then, through the wisdom of Chinese medicine, we are guided to orientate our understanding and our answers. As the author puts it, we are 'navigating a way forward that will provide relief and benefit the child'.

The book is underpinned by Rebecca's wealth of clinical experience as an acupuncture practitioner. It is written in a way that makes it accessible and useful for parents too. It shows how the Chinese medicine approach can help to relieve a child's anxiety or fear, soften their anger or worry, move stagnation or dampness, strengthen qi or blood and take care of sleep or food disorders.

The structure of the book is very clear and helpful. It begins with how to recognise imbalances of *qi*, *shen*, *jing* and blood and how these impact on a child's mental/emotional health. It then guides the reader to become familiar with the five basic constitutional types, their differing needs and the related different expressions of their troubled emotions.

Part 1, 'Understanding', provides examples of characteristics we can notice when children with a specific Element imbalance are thriving, or the emotional and relational difficulties they may have if they are struggling. In case we are still not clear, Rebecca gives us more clues by suggesting responses to issues such as 'What is the child's default "tired behaviour"? What motivates the child at school and in life in general? What is the child's cry when they are not happy?' And, in this last case, some examples may be: I'm bored. I'm worried. I'm not good enough. I'm scared. I'm fed up.

Part 2, 'Helping' discusses lifestyle, pointing out practical ways that parents and practitioners can support children's mental/emotional health through exercise, breathing, eating and sleeping habits; for example. I particularly liked her advice not to interpret any 'negative' emotion as a medical problem. Emotions are part of what makes us human. Rebecca also guides the reader to recognise when children need help. She suggests valuable ways to coax hidden emotions into the open, sit with them and soothe them.

The approach of starting from the individual child's emotional responses, rather than making assumptions, is supported by useful suggestions on how to be an 'emotion detective'. The skilled acupuncturist or concerned parent can look at the face and body language of a child and listen to the tone of their voice. I resonate deeply with the idea of feeling what emotions are evoked in ourselves while we are with the child. I would say that learning to identify how a patient's qi moves our qi is part of the diagnosis.

It is wonderful when we can be of help in smoothing a child's passage through thorny times and reinforcing their resilience when life is too difficult for them. Rebecca's excellent book provides both parents and practitioners with powerful tools to see when and how a child is troubled and gives them valuable tools to do something effective about it.

Elisa Rossi MD, Licensed Acupuncturist, 4-year PhD in
Clinical Psychology, Licensed Psychotherapist, BA in Philosophy

Acknowledgements

The process of writing a book always feels like a pregnancy, and this pregnancy has not been an entirely straightforward one. As it has progressed, there have been profound changes taking place in the world at large and in my own world. The birth of this book has been something that has kept me steady in the stormy seas of 2020. I have been hugely supported by family, friends and colleagues along the way and for that I am eternally grateful.

First and foremost, my husband, Peter Mole, deserves enormous thanks for his unwavering support throughout the process. Not only did he read every chapter and give me his valuable feedback, but he did it willingly and graciously. He also repeatedly picked up the domestic slack when I once again disappeared up to the attic to write. I could not have even contemplated embarking on this project, let alone completed it, without his love and support, which extends way beyond this book to everything I do in my life.

Equally deserving of a mention are my daughters, Alathea and Leyla, of whom I grow more proud each day. Despite the experience of having to share me with a previous book pregnancy still fresh in their minds, they did not hesitate for a second to declare their support this time. At the same time, they have been dealing with huge disruption in their own lives due to the COVID-19 pandemic and have showed the most astounding resilience and spirit. They bring more joy into my life, more smiles and laughter, than I would ever have imagined possible. Witnessing their astoundingly beautiful and wondrous selves blossom literally makes my heart swell with love. Thank you both for being you (and sorry if I have just embarrassed you!).

Many friends have helped the book come to fruition, in myriad ways. Jeannette Lichner was hugely instrumental in encouraging me to start this project and has always been there with support and advice during difficult moments along the way. Kanika Lang applied her sharp intelligence to some key chapters and her comments improved them. Moreover, the conversations we have on our walks not only feed my spirit but also help me enormously to clarify my thoughts. Special mention also needs to go to Darrell Nightingale who read almost the entire book with his unsurpassed attention to detail and let nothing slip past his Virgo eagle eyes. I am also hugely grateful to Adam Pearson. His encouragement and belief in me when I call and tell him of yet another hair-brained scheme is pivotal to my carrying them through. I am also grateful for him turning his Cornish home into a writing retreat for me and am sorry the pandemic put paid to that towards the end. My Aries-sister and long-term acupuncture buddy Soreh Levy gave invaluable help to come up with a title that finally felt right. Dr Michael Fitzpatrick helped me to refine my ideas about anxiety and depression, making many useful comments based on his wealth of experience as a general practitioner.

My colleagues Libby Temperley-Shell and Paloma Sparrow both generously offered to read parts of the book and gave valuable feedback. Andrew Wormald kindly contributed with his knowledge of Chinese characters. I am grateful to Sarah Hoyle who, once again, came up with just the illustrations I needed and is always a complete pleasure to work with.

Thanks also go to Maddy Budd and all the team at Singing Dragon. Their professionalism and efficiency makes them a joy to work with. I was able to hand over my 'baby' before the final part of the birthing process in the full knowledge that it would be looked after in the way I would want.

Each and every one of the children who come to the Panda Clinic for treatment inspires me and teaches me every day. Even when they are struggling and their lives feel difficult, they have the courage to show up and a willingness to put their faith in me and in Chinese medicine. Witnessing their struggles lessen and them beginning to once again enjoy life is truly the most rewarding work I can imagine. I have huge admiration for them and their families. Without them, this book would never have happened.

Finally, I would like to acknowledge parents and carers who stand alongside children whose mental/emotional health is struggling. There is no greater pain than witnessing a child or teenager suffering in this way. To all of you, I would like to extend my heartfelt compassion, support and encouragement. If this book helps even one of you to support a child to struggle less and thrive more, it will have been worth writing.

Notes for the reader
Case histories

I have changed the names and any other identifying features of the case histories which are dotted throughout the book.

Chinese medicine terms

In order to denote the use of a word in its Chinese medicine sense, I have used either an initial capital or italics. For example, if the word *blood* is italicised, it refers to the Chinese medicine concept of blood. If the word Fire has an initial capital, it refers to the Element of Fire.

Gender pronouns

I have alternated between female, male and gender-neutral pronouns throughout the book. I have attempted to do this in a balanced fashion and it is not my intention to favour any of them.

Introduction

As a paediatric acupuncturist, I spend my days with babies, children and teenagers who are all struggling. Sometimes this is because of a physical symptom. However, usually it is because the child is struggling with her mental/emotional health. I am writing this book because, time and time again, I see how applying the wisdom of Chinese medicine to a child's situation can bring about extraordinary change. It relieves the child's anxiety or lifts their mood. Chinese medicine contains so much insight that is timeless in its appeal and efficacy.

Getting behind the labels

'Anxiety' and 'depression' are terms or labels that are commonly used but which describe an extraordinarily vast array of different feeling states. A child may complain about feeling fearful, tense or worried. She may say she has negative thoughts, difficulty in concentrating or feels irritable much of the time. She may complain of a loss of appetite or having difficulty getting off to sleep. She may have low moods, or a lack of energy. She may say she feels tearful and no longer enjoys being around her friends and family. Parents may report that their child is withdrawn, grumpy, difficult or defiant, getting into trouble at school, or always squabbling with her siblings.

We may observe that she does not make eye contact or fidgets all the time. All of this may be casually labelled 'anxiety' and/or 'depression'. In order to help, the first thing to do is to put these labels to one side. As parents and practitioners, we need to listen to the child, observe her, explore (to the degree that she is able) what is going on in her internal world and gain an understanding of the context of her life. Although throughout the book you will see the terms 'anxiety' and 'depression', the focus is always on unpacking these convenient but limited labels.

The current state of childhood mental health

Not long ago, mental health problems in children were taboo or barely ever discussed. Nowadays, it can feel as if they have become almost fashionable. There are almost daily headlines about increased rates of child and teen anxiety, depression, self-harm and eating disorders.

By endlessly commenting on the rise of child and teen anxiety and depression, by calling it an epidemic, are we somehow magnifying the problem? Or, on the contrary, is it only now that we are finally as a society waking up to a problem that has been pushed under the carpet for too long?

Perhaps there is some truth in both these stances. Whichever way the truth lies, it is undeniable that there are vast numbers of children who struggle with their mental/emotional health.

What is normal?

In my clinic, I hear children of primary-school age talk about 'my anxiety', as if they regard it as being as much a part of who they are as the fact that they have brown hair or blue eyes. I hear teens announce that they need anti-depressants because their mood is low for a week or two around exam time. I also hear children saying that they feel anxious about feeling anxious, concerned that this means there is something wrong with them. I have seen adolescent mood swings and teenage heartbreak become medicalised. It is hard to escape the fact that it benefits pharmaceutical companies to pathologise more and more aspects of life.

Being fully human means feeling a wide range of emotions. Feeling anxious before starting a new school or low after you have lost a grandparent does not mean that you suffer from anxiety or depression. Nor does feeling fed up and angry at times when you are a teenager. However, it is a different matter when a child's feeling state begins to affect her everyday life, schooling and relationships. When a child's emotional world diminishes them and the lives of those around them, it is a sure sign of a pathology.

There is a fine line between turning every 'negative' emotion into a medical problem and ignoring the fact that a child needs help. However, it is a line that we as parents or practitioners must walk as carefully as we can. Both intervening prematurely and failing to act can exacerbate the problem.

Nature and nurture

It is an indictment of our society that so many of our young people are suffering. Yet we do not seem to have grappled sufficiently with the question of 'why?' There are, of course, too many children who grow up in crushing poverty or violent households, or with other problems in their life that understandably affect their moods and their emotional well-being. However, on the surface, the majority of children in the developed world today have it easy, compared with past generations. They have comfortable and warm houses, an abundance of food choices, and more clothes than they know what to do with, mostly attend more than good enough schools, have an astounding array of leisure activities available and have access to good-quality medical care.

Yet it is often these children whose mental/emotional health is suffering. They may not have to worry about their next meal, but their family may be under strain, their parents divorced, or they may feel enormous pressure to succeed in exams, look a certain way or have the right pair of trainers. The problems that 21st-century life causes for most children today are very different from those of a few generations ago, yet are pernicious enough to be causing huge amounts of unhappiness.

Chinese medicine understands that there are two aspects that need to be addressed. The first is the inherent nature of the child. Some children are born with more of a tendency to become anxious or feel low than others. It could be said that their mental/emotional constitution is somewhat weak. The second aspect with which we must be concerned is the child's lifestyle. It is the interaction between these two things that produces either a child who thrives or one who struggles.

There is little we can do to change a child's inherent nature. Yet what we can do is to try to recognise it and then to create a life for that child which, as far as possible, suits him. Chinese medicine, in particular the Five Element approach, is a wonderful tool to help both parents and practitioners understand the differences between children's emotional natures.

A child's lifestyle, on the other hand, is something that we do have some control over. There seems to be so much about the lifestyle of many children that makes it difficult for them to be happy, even for middle-class kids who seemingly have it all.

Rather than our focus being purely on the child and assuming that it is he who has or is 'the problem', we also need to look at the child's lifestyle and work out which aspects of it are preventing the child from thriving. There are aspects of life that are widely accepted as being normal and fine, but which compromise the mental/emotional well-being of many children.

There are, of course, some aspects of our children's lives that we cannot change. Most children will have times when life is difficult and does not go according to plan, or when they feel some pressure. Most will come across alcohol, drugs, social media and sexting at some point in their teenage years. Our role as parents or practitioners is to help a child develop the resilience to cope during these times, and to be able to manage better the parts of life that we are not able to change.

I make no apology for reminding people what we all surely already know: that having good connections with others, getting enough sleep, incorporating movement into daily life, etc., etc., are all essential for a child's mental/emotional well-being.

That this needs to be written is indicative of the fact that many children's early years no longer meet their basic needs. Many aspects of children's lives nowadays that are considered as the norm are often at the root of their problems. We scratch our heads and wonder why so many children are struggling, instead of noticing what is right in front of our eyes. Most of the time, creating solid mental/emotional health in our children is not rocket science. Part 2 of the book explores the key aspects of children's lives and how they can contribute to anxiety and depression.

What does Chinese medicine have to offer?

Chinese medicine is a lot more than acupuncture and herbalism. It is an entire philosophy and way of living. In order to help children, they do not necessarily need to be taken to a practitioner. The information contained in this book is all about adapting a child's lifestyle to suit her, so that her mental/emotional health can thrive.

Chinese medicine understands that the mind, the emotions and the body are one entity. It looks at the whole to understand what may be manifesting in one part. Sometimes, to help a child feel less anxious, the most effective approach is to make a change to her lifestyle that will, on the surface, primarily affect her physical body. For example, excessive exercise at too young an age could be detrimental not only to the child's body but also to her mental/emotional health. There is much to be gained from taking this holistic approach, rather than reducing our understanding of what is going on to levels of chemicals in the child's brain, or to a hormonal imbalance, for example.

The Chinese medicine system of the Five Elements provides a framework through which the differing natures and temperaments of children can be understood. It helps us to understand why each child's needs are unique. It also helps us to grasp the nuances of a child's mental/emotional state, once things have become imbalanced.

I know of no other system that so effectively helps us appreciate the fact that one child's medicine is another's poison, that one child's anxiety has a different flavour to it than another's, and that every child who has a low mood will experience that in her own unique way.

Part 1 of the book elucidates the Five Element model so that parents and practitioners can better understand children and the differing ways they manifest mental/emotional imbalance.

Filling a gap

Most children today who are significantly anxious and/or depressed are offered some kind of talking therapy as a first line of treatment, perhaps from a child psychologist or a cognitive behavioural therapist. While helpful for some, for many children talking therapy can be too direct and threatening. We know that the part of the brain that enables self-insight (the prefrontal cortex) does not fully develop until we reach our early twenties. This is why many children lack the maturity and insight that is needed to talk at length about their internal emotional world.

Those whose symptoms are more severe may be offered a range of medications, most commonly selective serotonin re-uptake inhibitors (SSRIs). SSRIs have side-effects and are often not licensed for use in children. Many parents have concerns about their child starting medication at such an early stage in their lives. Moreover, in many parts of the world, child and adolescent mental health services are hugely under-resourced at the same time as being inundated with the ever-increasing number of children who need help. There is often a waiting list of months, if not years, before a child can be seen.

The information contained in this book will empower parents to start making positive changes now. It can assist practitioners to guide both parents and children in order to make changes that will benefit children's mental/emotional health. These changes do not rely on pharmaceuticals or on the willingness of their child to talk to a therapist. Moreover, they are accessible to everybody because they do not cost money. Whether used alone or in conjunction with other interventions, Chinese medicine's unique perspective is a welcome additional approach to support children's mental/emotional well-being, which can be added to the rather limited existing ones.

Keeping the focus on the child

I have purposely chosen not to cite the wealth of medical research that has been done and continues to be done in the area of child and teen anxiety and depression. That research can be found in any number of articles and books on the subject. Much of what Chinese medicine has long since held to be important has lately been proven to be true by modern science.

This book encourages the reader not simply to do what a particular study suggests might be a good idea. It advocates observing the child, examining her life and navigating a way forward that will provide relief and benefit the child. While studies have their value, they can also divert us away from observing, understanding and responding to what is in front of us.

Long-term strategies in place of instant panaceas

This book does not offer a panacea that promises to cure every child's problems. Nor is it a manual full of yet another set of 'rules', which may suit one child but be detrimental to another. Although you will find many practical suggestions, it is not full of punchy sound bites, top tips or quick hacks. Creating an environment in which an individual child can thrive is a subtle and nuanced process, which can be challenging at times, and takes commitment. This book is an invitation to think differently.

It may challenge parents to let go of previously held notions about who their child is and what is right for them. Implementing the necessary changes may be difficult and may take time, but ultimately the potential benefits are manifold.

Finally, we cannot get away from the fact that what we are doing now societally is not working optimally for the young. Rates of child and teen anxiety and depression are rising, and the treatments on offer are of limited benefit. We have to do something differently if we are to stem the tide. This book is a call to arms.

The way forward is to understand and then accommodate the fact that each child has different needs. It is also to initiate changes to their lifestyle that can help them to thrive. Chinese medicine believes there is nothing more important than developing the art of 'nurturing the young'. In doing this, we not only create thriving children, but ones who will go on to have a much greater chance of becoming well-balanced adults.

Part 1

UNDERSTANDING

Chapter 1

Setting the Scene

The big picture

Before we dive in to talking about children's mental/emotional health, it is necessary to discuss a few key Chinese medicine concepts. These concepts will be referred to throughout the book, so you might want to check back to this chapter, as and when necessary, to refresh your understanding of them.

At first glance, concepts such as *yin/yang* can appear fairly easy to grasp. Many people find that the more they sit with these ideas, the deeper their understanding of them becomes. As you read and take on board these concepts, I hope that you will begin to *feel* and to *live* them rather than just have an intellectual understanding of them. Of course, in a book, words are the only vehicle to impart the nature of these ideas. My hope is that as you observe the children in your care and the world they live in, you will begin to see how these concepts are embodied.

I have been familiar with the language of Chinese medicine since 1995. The philosophy that underpins it endlessly reveals itself to me still, in ever different ways. For some readers, this will be their first encounter with the language of Chinese medicine. For others, these concepts will already be familiar. I hope that whichever is the case for you, the descriptions that follow will resonate and prove helpful.

Key Chinese medicine concepts

Chinese medicine is based upon a profound and extensive philosophy, a discussion of which could fill volumes on its own. Here I will limit my discussion to a brief, but I hope adequate, description of the key concepts that relate to childhood mental/emotional health. For anybody wishing to explore Chinese medicine further, I have listed some useful resources in the Bibliography at the end of the book.

The concepts we will discuss in this chapter are:

- a holistic medicine

- *yin/yang*

- the Five Elements.

A holistic medicine

You will likely have often heard Chinese medicine described as 'holistic'. This is a word that gets bandied about in many different contexts and is generally considered to mean treating symptoms within the context of the whole person, rather than isolating organs or parts of the body, as if they were just a cog in a machine.

In truth, any system of medicine can be practised more or less holistically, depending on the wisdom of the individual physician. However, what distinguishes Chinese medicine is that it places the diagnosis of the *person* at its very heart. It sees illness as a manifestation of an imbalance in the person. The illness or symptoms are often described as the 'branch', which stem from a deeper imbalance in the whole person, that is described as the 'root'. The great physician Sir William Osler said, 'Don't tell me what type of disease the patient has, tell me what type of patient has the disease.' His sentiments are very much in line with Chinese medicine, where the focus is on the person rather than the illness.

In our exploration of childhood anxiety and depression, our focus will be largely on the child and her constitutional nature, the circumstances of her life, and how the interaction between the two have led to her feeling anxious and/or depressed.

The body, mind and emotions are inseparable

Another aspect of the 'holistic' approach of Chinese medicine is that it views the mind, body and emotions as being one. What is meant by this is that anything that happens to the physical body will influence the mind and the emotions. Anything that happens in the child's emotional world will influence her mind and her body. Anything that happens in the child's mind will influence her physical body and her emotions.

It is an entirely Western construct, since the 1600s, to believe that the human body is little more than an extremely sophisticated machine, and that if there is a problem in one part then fixing that one part will solve the problem. Chinese medicine believes that the human body is much more than the sum of its chemistry and mechanics. That is why parts of the book focus on aspects of life that are generally believed to have more of an impact on the physical body than on the mental/emotional sphere, such as diet and exercise. In order to prevent and to heal anxiety or depression in a child, the entirety of the child needs to be in a state of health and functioning well. The mind and body are seen as an indivisible unit: a change in one often brings about a change in the other.

What does this mean in the real world?
What goes on in a child's body will influence her emotional state and her emotional state will influence what goes on in her body. It is easy to see this two-way relationship in action in children.

Here are a couple of examples:

THE THREE-YEAR-OLD WHOSE EYES ARE BIGGER THAN HIS STOMACH

Ralph goes to a birthday party and finds it hard to resist all the delicious foods that are on offer that he is not usually allowed to eat at home. He fills up on pizza, cake and biscuits, eating far more than he ever has done before. As a consequence, he gets a terrible stomach ache as this overload of food means his digestive system cannot cope. At the same time, his mood changes. He becomes grumpy and irritable. He gets annoyed with everything his mother says in the car on the way home. When he gets home, he throws a tantrum, screaming and shouting and throwing himself on the floor. Figure 1.1 illustrates this process.

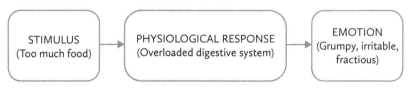

Figure 1.1 Bodily changes produce an emotion

THE ELEVEN-YEAR-OLD WHO WORRIES ABOUT SCHOOL

Maisie has to take an exam to get a place at her next school. She knows it is really important and is worried because she still does not really understand how to do the mathematics that she knows will come up in the exam.

She spends the whole of Sunday worrying about it and, as bedtime approaches, she finds she just cannot stop the worries from whirling around and around. As she tries to get to sleep, she develops a stomach ache. It is a dull, throbbing feeling that then makes dropping off to sleep even harder. Figure 1.2 illustrates this process.

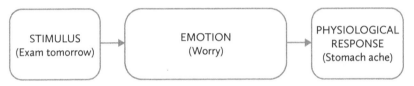

Figure 1.2 An emotion produces bodily changes

Yin/yang

The concept of *yin/yang* is probably the most important and distinctive theory underpinning Chinese medicine. *Yin/yang* represent opposite, but complementary, qualities. They are seemingly opposing forces, which are actually interconnected and interdependent. They give rise to each other and are interrelated. Together, *yin/yang* comprise the whole of creation. Figure 1.3 shows the famous *tai ji* symbol which illustrates *yin/yang* in perfect harmony; one flowing into another, *yin* containing *yang* and *yang* containing *yin*.

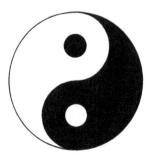

Figure 1.3 Tai ji symbol illustrating yin/yang

Each part of the *yin/yang* duality corresponds to certain phenomena, some examples of which are given below.

Yin   Rest, cold, descending, night-time, stillness, contraction, dark, passivity, decreasing, inwardness

Yang   Activity, heat, rising, daytime, movement, expansion, light, stimulation, increasing, outwardness

When a practitioner of Chinese medicine analyses a person's symptom or illness, she will think in terms of *yin/yang*. For example, she may explain a person's insomnia as being due to an excess of *yang* or their backache to a deficiency of *yang*. Or a person's fatigue may be due to an excess of *yin* or their agitation to a deficiency of *yin*. Illnesses, both physical and mental/emotional, arise as a result of, and are an expression of, an imbalance between *yin* and *yang*. Many of the suggestions given throughout this book are aimed at helping to redress the balance in a child between *yin* and *yang*.

Yin/yang in a child

In health, *yin/yang* will be in a state of equilibrium. A child will neither be too hot nor too cold. He will be active and energetic in the day, and sleep well at night. The concept of health in a child, however, is different to that in an elderly person. For example, we would expect a three-year-old to want to run around a lot more than a person in his eighties. This brings us to a key point, to which we will return again and again throughout the book:

Children are inherently abundant in yang.

This is what enables a child to grow and develop at an astonishing rate. Abundant *yang* is a sign of health in a child. However, it means that her needs are inherently different to that of an adult, who does not have such an abundance of *yang*. A healthy balance of *yin/yang* in a child is somewhat different to a healthy balance of *yin/yang* in an adult.

Yin/yang and mental/emotional health

As mentioned before, *yin/yang* needs to be in a state of equilibrium in order for a child to have strong mental/emotional health. We can use the lens of *yin/yang* as a way to start understanding the nature of poor mental/emotional health. For example, if a child tends towards feeling agitated and restless, it may mean that her *yin* is not quite robust enough. *Yin* helps a child to feel calm, restful and mentally robust. If, on the other hand, a child tends towards feeling low, unmotivated and lethargic, it may mean that her *yang* is insufficient. *Yang* enables a child to be joyful, motivated and energetic.

The key pathologies of *yin/yang* relevant to mental/emotional health, and which you will see throughout the book, are:

- *yin* deficiency

- *yang* deficiency.

Eight-year-old Solomon is typical of a '*yin*-deficient' child. His mum says he is *never* still. If he is not able to move around, he fidgets all the time. He takes a while to get off to sleep and also tends to wake early in the morning. He tosses and turns in his sleep and feels hot to the touch. He can easily become anxious. On the one hand, he seems to have boundless energy; on the other hand, he has dark circles under his eyes and, underneath his exuberance, his mum feels he is exhausted.

In contrast, his ten-year-old sister Jo is typical of a '*yang*-deficient' child. She can easily sleep for twelve or thirteen hours every night. She likes nothing more than to snuggle up on the sofa with a hot-water bottle and a book. It takes a lot of persuasion to get her to do any exercise. Her mum worries about her because, although she is extremely relaxed, she feels that she lacks spark and drive.

The Five Elements

Western culture talks of four elements, namely air, earth, fire and water. However, the Chinese system has five elements, each of which relates to a certain season (the fifth season being 'late summer' which, in the northern hemisphere, is approximately August and September). Figure 1.4 shows the Five Elements and related seasons.

Along with the concept of *yin/yang*, the Five Elements underpin the whole of Chinese medicine. They are the energetic foundations on which life is built. Each Element brings particular qualities to the world. For example, as you can see in Figure 1.4, the Wood Element is associated with the season of spring. In nature, spring is a time of rapid growth when vegetation bursts forth and the countryside becomes verdant. This is in contrast to winter, which is associated with the Water Element. Winter (and therefore the Water Element) is characterised by decline, stillness and hibernation.

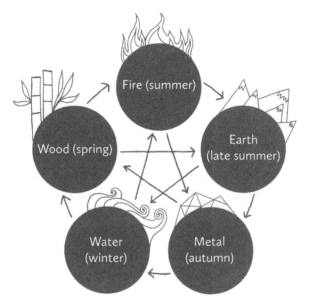

Figure 1.4 The Five Elements and related seasons

The Five Elements not only make up the natural world, but are also present within people. They can be thought of as the seasons within us, the different aspects that make up the complex beings that we are. For example, the part of a child that enables him to learn in school is different to the part that enables him to look after himself as he grows up. His drive to be with his friends as a teenager originates from a different part of him than his need to have a secure home life. On a day when he feels he could conquer the world, a different side of him is predominating than on a day when it feels hard to even turn up at school. Many of the key aspects of being human are associated with a different Element.

The Five Elements in children

During the first years of life, the Five Elements within a child are slowly maturing. The circumstances of a child's life, in combination with his innate nature, will influence how smoothly this maturation process happens.

In an ideal world (if there were such a thing), the growth and development of each Element within a child would be wholly supported by the events and circumstances of his early life. In reality, life is never quite ideal and the development of the Five Elements becomes distorted. Traumatic events, for example, prolonged separation from a parent or a serious illness, will obviously have an impact on a child's development.

However, less obvious aspects of life also influence the development of the Five Elements within a child. For examples, subtle dynamics within the family or having to move schools may be enough to create imbalance.

Particular aspects of life tend to affect a particular Element. For example, the quality of the relationships a child has in his life will predominantly (although not exclusively) impact his Fire Element. The degree to which he gets the nurture he needs will predominantly impact his Earth Element. Chapter 10, 'Family', discusses in more detail how the Elements are influenced by the dynamics of family life.

The Five Elements and emotions

We have already mentioned that each Element has a season associated with it. However, each Element actually has a group of 'associations', which have a similar quality of *qi* to the Element. Two of these associations are between physical organs and emotions. For example, the Water Element is associated with the Kidneys and the Bladder in the physical realm, and with the emotion of fear.

Earlier in this chapter, I described the way in which the body of a child affects her emotions and vice versa. Continuing with the example of the Water Element, if a child experiences fear, it may produce a physical symptom in her kidneys or bladder. A relatively common example of this is bed-wetting, which often (though not always) stems from a feeling of anxiety or insecurity. On the other hand, if a child has a bladder symptom it may produce the emotion of fear in her. For example, she may develop a bladder infection after swimming in a public pool. As well as the physical symptoms of the infection, she may also experience heightened fear or anxiety.

The Five Elements, the twelve channels and the organs

The Chinese medicine understanding is that there are twelve pathways of *qi* that travel through the body. Each is linked to an internal organ, and each organ is linked to one of the Five Elements. The Chinese medicine concept of an organ, however, is different to the Western concept. It incorporates much more than simply the physical structure.

In Chinese medicine, an organ is defined by its *function*. What it *does* is more important than what it *is*. For example, the Lungs are defined by the fact that they are responsible for the whole breathing process, from the nose, down the trachea and to the organ of the lungs themselves.

Even if an organ is removed, for example, the gall-bladder, the functioning of the channel and the *qi* relating to that organ remains. Table 1.1 illustrates the Five Elements and their associated Organs and emotions.[1]

Table 1.1 Five Elements, organs and emotions

ELEMENT	ORGANS	EMOTION
FIRE	HEART SMALL INTESTINE PERICARDIUM TRIPLE BURNER	JOY
EARTH	SPLEEN STOMACH	WORRY
METAL	LUNG LARGE INTESTINE	GRIEF
WATER	KIDNEY BLADDER	FEAR
WOOD	LIVER GALL-BLADDER	ANGER

The Five Elements and constitutional mental/emotional health

The notion that a child has a particular mental/emotional constitution (as well as a physical one) has been a part of Chinese medical philosophy for over 2000 years. But what does this actually mean? It conveys the idea of each child having a particular temperament or disposition, and having certain lifelong characteristics that may manifest in his psychological make-up. For example, parents describe how, from day one, a child has been prone to worry, or easy to anger. Parents who have more than one child are often struck by the different emotional and psychological tendencies of each of their children.

Chinese medicine understands that every child has a constitutional imbalance in one of the Five Elements. This means that the child tends to struggle with the smooth expression of the emotion connected with that Element. For instance, the emotion connected with the Fire Element is joy. A child with a constitutional imbalance in the Fire Element might find it hard to raise his joy, especially when he is on his own. Conversely, he might have a need to be constantly joyful, take on the role of the 'class clown' and avoid feeling emotions related to a lack of joy or sadness (which are, of course, a part of life).

Knowing in which Element a child's constitutional imbalance lies does not mean that we should start pigeon-holing a child. While every Fire child may share certain tendencies, each will also have a collection of unique traits. Knowing that a child's constitutional imbalance is Fire helps us to understand better what he might need, what he might find challenging, why he behaves in a certain way and how we can best support him.

We will look in more depth at the Five Elements in Chapters 4, 5 and 6. Chapter 4 will discuss how to recognise Five Element constitutional types, Chapter 5 will look at what each Element type needs in order to thrive, and Chapter 6 will look at how each Element type will manifest anxiety and depression in a different way.

So, what now?

We have now had a brief overview of these fundamental Chinese medicine principles. They will come alive throughout the book as we relate them to children and their mental/emotional health. Next, we will turn to some other key concepts, an understanding of which is essential before we go on to talk about anxiety and depression in more detail.

Endnote

1   You may notice that the Chinese system has two organs that are not considered as such in Western medicine, namely the Pericardium and the Triple Burner. The pericardium is the fibrous sheath that surrounds the heart. It is also sometimes known as the Heart-Protector. The Triple Burner has no physical location but is considered to have a regulating effect on all the other organs.

Chapter 2

What Children Are Made of: *Qi*, *Shen*, *Essence* and *Blood*

The big picture

In Chapter 1, we discussed the two most fundamental concepts, namely *yin/yang* and the Five Elements. This chapter describes the other key concepts that we will refer to throughout the book.

> While you may be eager to get on and read about the specifics of anxiety and depression, the rest of the book will be of more value and easier to use if you have previously read this chapter. You may also find it useful to check back to this chapter as you read on, in order to remind yourself of concepts that you come across later.

The Vital Substances

What are little boys made of?
What are little boys made of?
Snips and snails
And puppy-dogs' tails
That's what little boys are made of.

What are little girls made of?
What are little girls made of?
Sugar and spice
And everything nice
That's what little girls are made of.

While the nursery rhyme did not provide any sensible answers, it did ask an important question: 'What are children made of?' Chinese medicine understands that children are made of what are collectively known as 'the Vital Substances'. These are:

- *qi*

- *shen*

- *essence*

- *blood.*

These four substances are the building blocks of a child's body and mind. We will now discuss them in detail.

Qi

Like *yin/yang* and the Five Elements, the concept of *qi* (pronounced 'chee') also lies at the heart of Chinese medicine. It is very difficult to find an adequate translation of the word. Many have been proposed, such as 'energy', 'material force', 'vital energy' and 'matter'. The reason *qi* is so difficult to translate is that it is fluid in nature. *Qi* can manifest in different forms and be different things in different situations. For this reason, I have chosen not to translate it but simply to use the word *qi* throughout the book.

Qi is a kind of life 'energy' that exists in everything in the world that we would think of as being alive. *Qi* flows through a child's body, is constantly changing, has its own rhythms, cycles and movements. *Qi* is affected by a child's external environment, for example, the weather, the seasons, the emotions of those around her. It is also affected by the child's internal landscape, for example, her emotions, how fast she is growing, what she eats. *Qi* is consumed by activity, and replenished by air, food and rest.

Eastern exercises such as *tai qi* or *qi gong* are methods of trying to harness and balance one's *qi*. The equivalent concept in the Hindu tradition is *prana*. *Prana* can be developed or balanced by the practice of yoga. Some basic observations of any children you know can, even to the untrained eye, reveal a lot about the *qi* of children. For example, a child who never tires, makes her presence felt as soon as she enters a room and has a healthy appetite may be described as having strong *qi*. In contrast, a child who easily tires, tends to let other children take the lead and is picky about food may be described as having weak *qi*.

It is hard not to interpret words like 'strong' and 'weak' as being either good or bad. Our Western minds like to categorise things in this polarised way. In reality, there are advantages and disadvantages to having both strong *qi* and weak *qi*. The most important thing is that parents, carers and, as they grow, children themselves should recognise and accept each child's unique nature and live accordingly.

Just as with *yin/yang*, the state of a child's *qi* determines the state of her health; conversely, the state of her health affects the state of her *qi*.

Qi in a child

There are some important and particular characteristics which are specific to the child's *qi*. First, the child's *qi* is said to be fragile. This means that it is not yet fully developed, and is therefore more easily influenced by what happens to it. The child's *qi* can be likened to an undercooked cake. If you touch it, it will be likely to collapse and perhaps leave a mark. In contrast, a fully cooked cake will likely just spring back when you touch it.

Another characteristic of the child's *qi* is that it becomes very easily unstable. It does not take much for the flow and rhythm of the child's *qi* to go awry. You can see this in action when a toddler becomes quickly very upset. Her body may shake, she may cry inconsolably and only begin to settle with the soothing presence of a trusted adult. The child may not be able to regain her equilibrium on her own but needs an external source of help.

As mentioned above, every child will have slightly different *qi*. Rather than treating every child the same and expecting the same of all children, the key to raising a child with good mental/emotional health is to respond to who she is.

Qi and mental/emotional health

Imbalances in *qi* can be a contributory factor in some cases of childhood anxiety and depression. For example, if a child's *qi* is not flowing properly – what we usually term being 'stagnant' – it can lead to a low mood and a feeling of hopelessness. If a child's *qi* is rather weak, it can mean she has a propensity to be easily knocked off-kilter by relatively small life events.

The key pathologies of *qi* relevant to anxiety and depression, and which you will see throughout the book, are:

- *qi* stagnation

- *qi* deficiency

- counterflow *qi* (*qi* rebelling upwards).

Fourteen-year-old Rachel has a tendency to *qi* stagnation. Her younger brother describes her as 'grumpy and moody'. He says, 'You never know which Rachel you are going to get.' One day she is happy and joyous; the next she walks around with a dark cloud over her head. Sometimes she runs upstairs shouting and slams her bedroom door, and nobody in the family knows quite what has upset her. Her moods have definitely improved since she has started cycling to and from school, rather than taking the bus. This is typical of *qi* stagnation, in that the symptoms tend to improve with movement.

Shen

Shen is perhaps one of the most elusive of all the Chinese medicine concepts, but also the most central to any discussion of mental/emotional health. It is usually translated as either 'mind' or 'spirit', but both of these are inadequate. *Shen* encompasses a range of different Western terms and ideas, including:

- mental health

- emotional health

- cognitive function

- spirit and vitality.

As it is so hard to translate adequately, throughout the book I will use the word *shen*.

As well as *qi*, *shen* determines a child's emotional resilience. It is also the part of a child that makes her truly unique. *Shen* enables a child, as she grows, to reveal her uniqueness and her true nature to the world and live according to it. The sinologist Claude Larre described *shen* like this: 'The *shen* are that by which a given being is unlike any other; that which makes an individual an individual more than a person.'[1]

It's worth pausing for a moment and reflecting on that statement. We would all say that of course we *know* that every child is different and needs to be treated accordingly. However, it is all too easy merely to pay lip service to that truth. A combination of our own *shen*, our history and the pressures of our lives may result in our relating to children on the basis of various assumptions about who they are and what they need. The more we relate from a place of curiosity rather than assumption, the more we create space for the *shen* of the child to flourish.

Shen and children

The *shen* of a child is especially delicate. It is not firmly 'rooted', which means it can be easily thrown off balance. This is why a child is so strongly influenced by her emotional environment and also why her emotions may easily become intense and overwhelming.

Shen and mental/emotional health

The *shen* is absolutely fundamental to a child's mental/emotional health. The *shen* determines how emotionally resilient she may be. The nature of a child's *shen* explains why one child may feel devastated by a rejection from a friend for months, while another gets up, brushes herself off and starts making new friends. Once again, there is a reciprocal relationship. The *shen* will determine a child's response to events in her life; events in her life will impact the *shen*. When a child feels anxious or depressed over a period of time, it is a sure sign that her *shen* has become imbalanced.

The *shen* becomes imbalanced in the following different ways:

- *shen* disturbance
- *shen* deficiency
- *shen* clouded.

Each of these types of *shen* pathology may be involved in anxiety and depression, and you will see references to them throughout the book.

Nine-year-old Leon has some *shen* disturbance. He becomes very anxious in the evening and struggles to get off to sleep. His teachers have noticed that it is difficult for him to concentrate in lessons. He begins talking to other children and cannot stop when asked.

Six-year-old Alma has a deficient *shen*. She is extremely shy, and barely ever interacts with other children in her class. She struggles to make eye contact with her teachers or her peers. She is extremely sensitive and becomes very easily upset by the words or actions of another child.

Seven-year-old Zac has a clouded *shen*. His parents and teachers describe him as being 'in a world of his own'. He seems quite contented but very often is so engrossed in his fantasy world that he appears not to hear what people are saying to him or to be aware of what is going on in his surroundings. It is hard to connect with him and he seems to lack the usual emotional responsiveness of a child of his age.

Essence

Essence, a translation of the Chinese term *jing*, describes a substance that is the foundation of a child's physical life and health. It is often compared to the Western concept of genes or DNA. It is the very fabric of a child's physical body.

Pre-birth and post-birth *essence*

A child inherits what we call pre-birth *essence* from her mother and father. There is little that can be done to change pre-birth *essence*. The *essence* she is born with is the *essence* she has. A child may be born with extremely robust and strong *essence*, or *essence* which is not so strong. A child with poor *essence* will need to live his life more mindfully in order to avoid becoming ill than one who was born with strong *essence*. In a poker game, if you are dealt a hand of low cards, it is even more important that you play skilfully than for a player who was dealt a hand of high cards.

However, pre-birth *essence* is also nourished by post-birth *essence*. Post-birth *essence* depends on food, fresh air and the balance of rest and activity in a child's life. So there is a lot that can be done to optimise a child's post-birth *essence*. The better the post-birth *essence*, the less the pre-birth *essence* will be taxed. Pre-birth *essence* is like a child's savings account and post-birth *essence* is like her current account. If a child can be helped to live within her means, and not have to withdraw from her savings account, it will help her to live a longer and, most importantly, a healthier life.

Seven-year-old Noreen had always reached her developmental mile-stones slightly later than her peers. She caught every bug that was going around and seemed to suffer more acutely and take longer to get over them than other children. By the end of each school term, she was so exhausted she could barely function. The only time she seemed to really thrive was during the long summer holidays, when she was under no pressure and felt at her most vital in the warm, sunny weather. Noreen was typical of a child with weak *essence*.

Essence underpins growth and development

Essence is also pivotal in determining how well a child grows and develops. If she repeatedly misses key developmental milestones, we may suspect that she has insubstantial *essence*. Being the very fabric of a child's physical make-up, *essence* can be described as containing a child's developmental coding, making sure that the right thing happens at the right time.

For example, a child will usually start walking around the age of one, stringing a few words together around eighteen months and have all her milk teeth by about 30 months. There is a huge range of what can be considered 'normal', but if a child is dropping significantly behind in several of these milestones, it points to a problem with her *essence*.

Essence governs the cycles of life

Chinese medicine understands that humans have distinct cycles of growth and development. These cycles are said to be of seven years' length in girls and women, but of eight years in boys and men. So, around the age of seven, a girl will transition to a new phase of development, as she will again at around the age of fourteen and so on throughout her life. One of the most recognised of these transitions from one cycle to the next is puberty. These transitions are crucial times. *Yin/yang* are in a state of flux. Depending on what happens in a child's life, she may either throw off a pre-existing health problem or it may become more entrenched. These cyclical transitions can be either a time of crisis or an opportunity. I will discuss this in more detail in Chapter 11.

Essence in a child

Childhood is a time when a child's *essence* gradually emerges, matures and reveals itself. When a baby is conceived, her completely unique *essence* starts to form. After birth and throughout childhood, the seeds will gradually germinate, and then start to grow and eventually blossom. A parent's job is to provide a satisfactory environment for this process to take place.

Essence and mental/emotional health

From what you have read so far, it might be hard to see the connection between *essence* and mental health. However, as you will see time and again throughout this book, it is impossible to separate a child's physical state from her mental/emotional one. What goes on in the body affects the mind and vice versa.

● If you are reading this thinking that it sounds as if some children are just plainly disadvantaged by having a poor constitution, it might be helpful to change your perspective. There are, of course, some children who are dealt a bad hand. These children are plagued by poor mental/emotional or physical health even if they live an exemplary life. However, they are few and far between.

A child with, for example, extremely weak *essence* may flounder if he is expected to live the hectic life that his peers enjoy. On the other hand, he may thrive if he is able to live a quieter life that better suits his nature.

As parents and practitioners, we need to support a child to find a path in life which is right for him, based on his individual nature and constitution. This does not mean that we can create the ideal situation for every child but that we need to change the aspects of his life that it is possible to change and support the child to deal, as best as he can, with those aspects that cannot be changed.

> Chinese medicine speaks of *essence, qi* and *shen* as 'the Three Treas-
> ures'. *Essence* is the source of life; *qi* activates *essence*; and *shen* gives
> both *essence* and *qi* spirit. The state of one is dependent on and
> influenced by the state of the other. In this book, we are mainly con-
> cerned with issues of the *shen*. However, *essence* and *qi* are relevant
> because of the impact they have on the *shen* and the impact of the
> *shen* upon them.

Blood

Blood is another manifestation of *qi*. It is a *yin* substance which circulates
continuously throughout the body. However, beyond that, the Chinese medicine characteristics of *blood* are different from the red fluid of Western
medicine. As we are concerned here with mental/emotional health, I shall
limit my discussion of *blood* to its relevance in that sphere.

Blood and mental/emotional health

Blood can be understood as an anchor for a child's emotions. It has a grounding and rooting influence. Chinese medicine talks about *blood* 'housing' the
emotions. Without a house, a child's emotions may float around and she may
become disconnected from them. She may feel that her emotions are out
of her control and they may begin to dominate. For example, at bedtime, a
child may find her worries go around and around in her mind and she cannot
switch them off. This might be because her *blood* is not strong enough to
anchor them.

Like *yin*, *blood* also provides a degree of emotional consistency and resilience. When *blood* is weak or deficient, a child may feel emotionally sensitive
or vulnerable. She may find she easily becomes tearful. *Blood* deficiency can
also create a low-level agitation, although this is not usually as strong as the
agitation that comes from *yin* deficiency.

Blood tends to come into the picture in terms of mental/emotional health
problems around puberty, and is especially relevant for girls. When a girl begins menstruation, and especially if she bleeds heavily, her *blood* may become
weak and this may have an impact on her emotions as described above. This
will be discussed in further detail in Chapter 11, 'Times of Change'. It is also
common for children who have an insufficiently considered vegetarian diet

to have weak *blood*. This will also be discussed further in Chapter 16, 'What to Eat'.

The key pathology of *blood* relevant to mental health, and which you will see throughout the book, is *blood* deficiency.

Fifteen-year-old Susan has started to feel increasingly anxious over the last year, since she began menstruating. Her anxious thoughts tend to take hold in the evening, especially when she is tired. She finds as she gets closer to bedtime, her thoughts start going around and around in her head. She is also finding it harder to concentrate for long periods on her school work and finds she is just staring at the words without really taking anything in. She cries more easily than she used to and gets quite agitated by all the banter on social media. The way Susan feels is typical of someone with *blood* deficiency.

Bringing the theory to life

Having read about the key Chinese medicine concepts related to mental/emotional health, try to observe them in action. Be curious about the differing natures of the children you know. Here are some questions you might want to ponder whenever you are around children:

▶ With a particular child in mind, reflect on whether you think he has strong or weak *qi* (remembering that one is not 'better' than the other). What has led you to your answer?

▶ Think of two children of a similar age and make a mental note of their differences. Does this tell you anything about the nature of their *qi*, *shen*, *essence* or *blood*? If so, what?

▶ Do you know of a teenage girl who has struggled more with her emotions since beginning menstruation? If so, do you think she is *blood* deficient? What might make you think this?

▶ Do you know of any children who you think have relatively weak *essence*? If so, what makes you think this? And is the nature of their daily life taking this into account?

So, what now?

We have now covered all the key principles and concepts of Chinese medicine related to our discussion of childhood anxiety and depression. Before we move on to looking at the different Element types, we will take a brief look at how Chinese medicine understands the nature of children and childhood in general.

Endnote

1   C. Larre and E. Rochat de la Vallée (1986) *Survey of Traditional Chinese Medicine* (Paris: Institut Ricci), p. 164.

Chapter 3

The Nature of Children and Childhood

The big picture

In order to understand how and why a child becomes anxious or depressed, we first need to understand the nature of childhood. Chinese medicine has many insights into how a child is inherently different to an adult. Due to this perspective, paediatrics has been a specialty of Chinese medicine for over 2000 years.

These insights arose out of observations of children in everyday life. They did not come from research done in a laboratory. Neither were they expounded by academics or scientists who had little direct experience of babies and children. They are at the same time incredibly simple yet deeply profound. They are often insights that we instinctively know to be true, yet which we ignore. They remind us to look not at how many millilitres of milk a baby has drunk but at whether she appears sated and comfortable. They remind us to focus not solely on the temperature showing on the thermometer but also on the state of the child.

Nurturing the young

Approximately 1400 years ago, one of Chinese medicine's most famous doctors, Sun Simiao, wrote that 'There is no *dao* [meaning "skill" or "practice"] among the common people that is greater than the *dao* of nurturing the young. If [children] are not nurtured when they are young, they die before reaching adulthood.'[1]

Sun Simiao was writing at a time when infant mortality rates were much higher than they are now, at least in the developed world, hence using what reads to us as rather alarmist language. Yet so much of what he said about how to 'nurture the young' is relevant to 21st-century children. This is the subject of Part 2, when we will discuss in detail the kind of lifestyle advice that helps to prevent and heal childhood anxiety and depression.

Venerating the root

Sun Simiao also spoke of 'venerating the root'. He had a deep understanding of the fact that if we take care of the beginnings of life, we lay good foundations for the rest of life. This is why it is of such crucial importance that we do everything we can to address anxiety and depression in children. Anxious and/or depressed children are much more likely to go on to be anxious and/or depressed adults. By finding ways to help a child feel better when she is young, we not only improve the quality of her childhood but we potentially improve the quality of the rest of her life.

Three phases of influence

A child's mental/emotional health is influenced by three factors:

- his constitution

- his time *in utero*

- the care in and circumstances of infancy and childhood.

There is nothing that can be done about constitution or, after the event, what happens during pregnancy. However, the area where we can make an enormous difference is in the way we care for a child in his early life. Part of that care also means doing what we can to create circumstances in which a child is most likely to be able to thrive. In order to do that, we must first understand the characteristics of children. In Chapter 4, we will look at ways to understand the differences between children. Before we do that, however, we will focus on the characteristics which are common to all children.

Common characteristics of children
Children are strongly impacted by their environment

A young child can be likened to a seedling. He is delicate, fragile and vulnerable to his surroundings. We would never think of planting a seedling in a cold and unprotected environment, but would first nurture it in a greenhouse, which provides warmth and protection. In the same way, a child needs to be protected in the first weeks, months and years of life. As he grows more robust, he becomes more able to withstand a less protected environment.

In one sense, nurturing a child is all about an appropriate and ever-changing balance of nurture and protection on the one hand, exposure and independence on the other hand. In an ideal world, a child will receive large amounts of nurture and protection in early life, and a gradually increased amount of freedom and independence as she grows. Many children experience the opposite. They may have an excessive amount of separation in the early years, followed by too much restriction and a lack of freedom in the later years.

The right balance between protection and exposure will vary from child to child. It is important to point out that we need not aim for perfection in this regard, and that a reasonable balance will suffice.

On the one hand, if a child is strongly over-protected, it will not allow him a chance to develop mental/emotional resilience. Psychologists talk of a concept of 'stress inoculations', meaning that small amounts of short-term stress help a child to produce what we might term 'mental/emotional antibodies'. From the Chinese medicine point of view, if the different aspects of a child – the Five Elements, *qi*, *yin/yang*, *blood* – do not get used and activated, they will not become robust and strong.

On the other hand, if a child is not adequately protected from his environment and does not receive enough nurture in his early years, his process of growth and development may be impaired or interrupted. Some experiences or traumas are not able to be absorbed and assimilated and may leave a permanent marker on a child's mental/emotional health.

Children are like sponges

As well as being vulnerable to their environment, children are also like sponges that absorb the atmosphere in their surroundings, which is a manifestation of *qi*. As such, it has a particular quality to it. In particular, emotions lend a distinct quality to the atmosphere. Most children sense any strong emotion in those they are with, even when the emotion is not overtly expressed. If a child spends the day in a classroom with a tense and stressed-out teacher, he will often come home feeling tense and stressed out himself. If he lives with a mother who is sad, or a father who is fearful, he may find himself feeling sad or fearful.

On a temporary basis, this is relatively unproblematic. However, when it becomes an ongoing situation it can have a long-term impact. Chinese medicine understands that a child is delicate and malleable when she is young, and gradually becomes firmer and more 'set' as she grows. An emotion which a child is exposed to over a period of months or years becomes imprinted on her, like a footprint left in wet cement that will remain as the cement dries. Many aspects of childhood, as we will see, leave a kind of energetic imprint on the child's balance of *yin/yang* and on their Vital Substances.

Hayley is a bright and articulate woman in her twenties. She had always struggled with high levels of anxiety and, despite a lot of reflection, could never quite get to the bottom of *why* this was. She felt that she had not had any particularly difficult things happen to her in her life so far. It was only when she left home, and had some separation from her parents, that she gained some clarity. When she went back to visit her parents after a few months of being away, it struck her how highly anxious her mother was. She had become so used to this as a child that she just thought it was normal. Hayley believes that as a child she simply absorbed her mother's anxiety and that it had become her own. Having brought this connection to light, and with the help of some therapy and acupuncture, her anxiety levels dropped significantly. Although it remained something she needed to work on, her quality of life greatly increased.

Childhood is characterised by rapid growth and development

It is stating the obvious to say that childhood is characterised by rapid growth and development. However, this is highly significant in how we care for children. A child's resources need to be available to support her growth and development. If they are diverted to meeting the needs of a demanding or stressful life, then something will have to give. According to Chinese medicine, the first seven or eight years of life, but to some degree the years up until a child stops growing, should primarily be concerned with building foundations. Just as we would not think about building walls or a roof or decorating a house before having laid a solid foundation, so it should be with a child. If a child is given an opportunity to use her internal resources to build a solid base of physical, mental and emotional health, it will pay dividends for the rest of her life.

One of my Chinese medicine teachers used a lovely analogy to explain how we need to care for children. He described how if we plant a young tree in the ground, our focus should be on creating the right environment in which the tree can grow. We should make sure that the soil has good nutrients, that it is well watered and that the tree is not overshadowed by other, bigger trees. Having made sure that the environment is conducive to growth, we would then allow the tree to grow in the way that is natural to it.

This is how Chinese medicine understands we should approach the care of children. Our focus should be very largely on the environment we create for them, rather than being overly concerned to influence the way the child's personality develops. Every child has their own unique, inherent potential and our job as parents is to create an environment in which that potential can reveal itself and flourish.

Children are abundant in *yang* and have immature *yin*

In Chapter 1, we discussed the fundamental Chinese medicine concept of *yin/yang*. We will now delve a little deeper and look at how this relates to children.

Children are described as having a 'pure *yang*' constitution. They are the very essence of *yang*. This is what enables them to grow and develop so quickly. It also means they have a great need to run around and to be active in order to not become 'stagnant'. Most parents of a young child know that there will come a point in the day when they have to send their child outside to let off steam. The abundant enthusiasm and inquisitiveness that are characteristics of most young children are also expressions of their exuberant *yang*.

This abundant *yang* also has relevance to the mental/emotional health of a young child. *Yang* has an upwards, outwards motion and will easily feel stifled if it is constrained. So a young child needs to be allowed to express this *yang*, not only through physical movement but through emotional expression. He may have intense feelings which arise quickly and have a lot of force behind them. If he is given the message that this is somehow 'wrong', it can lead to his natural exuberance being repressed, which may eventually have a negative impact on his mental/emotional well-being.

In contrast, a child's *yin* is not yet fully developed and therefore is often referred to as 'immature'. *Yin* has a downwards, inwards and contracting motion. As it is undeveloped, it means it does not easily hold down the exuberant *yang*, which then has a tendency to rise upwards to the child's head. This rising *yang* is involved in many mental/emotional, behavioural and physical conditions commonly seen in children, including anxiety. Throughout the book, we will discuss aspects of life that can help to nourish the *yin* of a child and therefore lessen this tendency of *yang* to rise up.

Adolescence is characterised by a surge in *yang*

It is not only young children who have an abundance of *yang*, however. *Yang* always surges to fuel any time of rapid growth and development. Adolescence, specifically puberty, is another such time. At this time, *yang* also fuels the strong drive that teenagers have towards independence and to separate psychologically from their parents and family.

While this surge of *yang* is necessary, it can also create problems. It can mean that feelings and tendencies that have previously been bubbling away under the surface now become more pronounced. This is why anxiety, for example, becomes more common in the teenage years. It is as if the *yang* magnifies emotions that were previously only subtle. Of course, some emotions that arise during the teenage years are completely new to the child. Even when that is the case, they are often very strongly felt because of the abundance of *yang* that characterises this time.

So, to summarise

▸ Children are strongly impacted by their environment.

▸ Children are like sponges, absorbing the atmosphere in their surroundings.

▸ Because children grow and develop so rapidly, they have limited resources available to deal with a stressful or overly busy life.

▸ Children have an abundance of *yang* and immature *yin*. This means they have a great need to express themselves but also a propensity for emotions to become intense and overwhelming.

So, what now?

Having looked at characteristics that *all* children have in common, we will now look at what makes children *different* to each other, and how to give different children different care.

Endnotes

1   S. Wilms (trans.) (2015) *Venerating the Root: Part 2*. Sun Simiao's *Bei Ji Qian Jin Yao Fang*, Volume 5: Paediatrics (Corbett, OR: Happy Goat Productions), p. xviii.

Chapter 4

Nature: Five Element Constitution

The big picture

Chinese medicine understands that every one of us is born with a different mental/emotional nature. This is related to which of the Five Elements is more imbalanced than the other four. Every child will have one Element that is her 'Achilles heel'. Just as a child may be prone to headaches or digestive upsets, she will also be prone to particular feeling states based on her elemental imbalance. A child with a constitutional imbalance in the Fire Element, for example, may be prone to feeling unloved whereas a child with a constitutional imbalance in the Wood Element may be prone to feeling angry. A Fire child will, of course, feel a wide range of emotions, but feeling unloved will be a state she most easily falls into when she is not thriving. While she will convey many different transient emotional states at different times, feeling unloved may be her fundamental or recurrent emotional tendency.

Knowing and understanding a child's elemental imbalance is a wonderful way of supporting his mental/emotional health. It enables us to understand the reasons behind a child's challenging behaviour, to recognise *why* a child may struggle in one area of life and to know *what* it is he most needs from us in order to thrive. It enables us to get to the nub of the issue and put our focus where it is most needed.

Becoming an Element detective

Chinese medicine practitioners focus on certain outward signs to diagnose which of the Five Elements is a person's constitutional type. These include the tone of the voice, the subtle colours around a person's eyes and mouth, her body odour and the emotion she has most difficultly expressing smoothly. This is an art in which it takes years to become competent.

The approach I suggest in this book is focused more on looking at behaviour. While this may be a less refined way of diagnosing an elemental imbalance, it is one that is accessible to parents and non-Chinese medicine practitioners. However, behaviour is always a response to an underlying feeling or energetic state. I therefore urge the reader to constantly be asking himself what is *underneath* a behaviour.

For example, let's take a common scenario of a teenager who is spending all his time in his bedroom and avoiding communicating with his family. This behaviour could have many underlying causes. It could be that the teenager is angry, and hiding away means he can avoid having to deal with this uncomfortable emotion. For another, it could be that he is anxious, and he stays in his room to avoid situations that trigger his anxiety. The key issue is not the fact that he is staying in his room but *why* he is staying in his room.

The behaviours described in the book that are typical of different Element types are therefore suggestions and indicators. They are meant as a guide to understanding a child. However, the best way to gain understanding is to observe the child. So, having read this chapter, I encourage the reader to put the book aside, to sit with and absorb the information and then to put it out of their head and become a keen observer. Confucius said, 'It is better to listen with your mind than listen with your ears but better still is to listen with your *qi*. The ears only record sounds, the mind can only analyse and categorise but the *qi* is empty and receptive.'[1]

Behavioural spectra

Each Element has certain emotions and behaviours associated with it. When the Element is in balance, a child's emotions and behaviour patterns are also balanced. When the Element is out of balance, related emotions and behaviours are at one end of a spectrum or the other. For example, the emotion connected with the Fire Element is joy. A child whose Fire Element is out of balance may at times be lacking in joy and at other times be excessively joyful. She may oscillate between one end of the spectrum and the other but struggle to find a steady place in the middle.

Getting to the root of the problem

It is important to remember that, although every child will have a constitutional imbalance in just one Element, she will also contain aspects of the other four Elements. Furthermore, the Five Elements are all connected in such a way that, when one is imbalanced, it will create some degree of imbalance in each of the other four.

This can mean that, as you read this chapter, you may find yourself thinking, 'I can see something of every Element's description in my child.' The objective is to try to look deeper than passing appearances. Your child may have become angry today, but would you really describe her as 'an angry child'? Your child may look after her little brother well when she is asked, but does she live for looking after others? Your child may have lots of friends but does being around them really change her demeanour?

A final word of caution

Giving a child a Five Element 'type' should not be about pigeon-holing him. If there were a room with one hundred Wood children in, for example, each child would of course be completely unique. However, they would be likely also to share certain similar characteristics. I therefore also urge readers not to get into thinking, 'Little Johnnie is a Wood child, therefore he will be feeling this,' or 'Little Johnnie is a Wood child, so he will respond like that.' Little Johnnie may well be a Wood child, but he is also completely unique. The descriptions that follow should be used as a guide to understanding a child but should never be used in place of observing and responding to the individuality of every child.

Fire

A thriving Fire child

When a child with a Fire constitutional imbalance is thriving, you may notice that the following qualities or characteristics stand out in him:

- He is very loving towards others.

- He has a sparkle that make others want to be around him.

- He oozes radiance and vitality.

- He tends to be optimistic and enthusiastic.

- He is warm and sensitive.

- He is adept at connecting with others.

- He navigates different types of relationships with ease.

- He is robust and resilient against life's knocks.

- He maintains a relatively constant level of joy.

A struggling Fire child

When a child with a Fire constitutional imbalance is struggling, he may have particular difficulties in the following areas:

Relationships

- He may feel very easily hurt and rejected, and struggle to get over a rejection.

- He may dive too quickly into friendships, rather than going through the appropriate steps to gradually create intimacy.

- He may have a desperate need for contact with others and struggle to be on his own in an age-appropriate way.

- He may cut himself off from others and avoid intimacy because he feels too vulnerable.

- He may struggle to make eye contact (because he feels so vulnerable).

Expression of joy

- He may appear chronically lacking in joy, as if he has lost his smile.

- He may be compulsively cheerful and avoid sad feelings at all cost. He is the class or family clown, which may be attractive, but it is compulsive.

- He may laugh inappropriately, especially when talking about something sad.

- His moods may be very changeable, constantly going between joyful and sad but rarely finding a happy but calm place in the middle.

Other signs of a Fire child

- He will light up when he is given warmth. He cannot fail to be moved by this, whereas for another child it may not bring about a change in his mood.

- His voice may at times sound flat and rather lacking in joy.

- He may at times lack any kind of red hue to his complexion, especially by the sides of his eyes.

Lola has a constitutional imbalance in the Fire Element. She is at her happiest when she is surrounded by her group of close friends, who mean everything to her. When she is with them, she is often gregarious and the one making the others laugh. On the other hand, when she is with people she does not know so well, she can be noticeably shy and quiet. Her parents are aware that she struggles when they and the rest of the family are busy and distracted. She can moan and complain that she is bored if she is not getting anybody's full attention. She does not like it when somebody else in the family is low, and naturally takes on the role of trying to cheer everybody up.

Earth
A thriving Earth child

When a child with an Earth constitutional imbalance is thriving you may notice that the following qualities or characteristics stand out in him:

- He is exceptionally good at caring for and empathising with others.

- His friends and classmates often turn to him for support.

- He is very secure and grounded in himself.

- He is adept at looking after his own needs.

- He is able to separate from his parents in an age-appropriate way.

- He has a healthy appetite and relationship with food.

- He has good concentration and focus.

A struggling Earth child

When an Earth child is struggling, he may have particular difficulties in the following areas:

- He is excessively dependent, needy and/or clingy.

- He has a seemingly endless need for sympathy (an empty well that can never be filled).

- He has a tendency to take on the weight of the world.

- He is prone to worry and overthinking.

- He feels it is his responsibility to help and support everybody.

- He has an unhealthy relationship with food (he comfort eats, controls his eating or stops eating when stressed, for example).

- He struggles to concentrate.

- His voice may at times have a lilt to it, almost as if he were singing.

- He may at times have a yellow hue to the side of his eyes and around his mouth.

Jamie has a constitutional imbalance in the Earth Element. He is soft and caring, and the one in his friendship group in whom others naturally confide. They all perceive him to be a good listener and always willing to offer sympathy and advice. His parents notice that when he is ill, compared with his siblings, he needs enormous amounts of sympathy and care. His mum said that when he is tired or worried about something, she can feel quite drained by the degree of neediness he displays. This is at odds with his usual stoic nature. He is a hard worker and has the ability to concentrate really well. He does tend to worry a lot about his work.

Both Fire and Earth types tend to be 'people persons'. Whereas Fire types tend to be looking for and giving love and warmth, Earth types tend to be looking for and giving care and support. The drive for a Fire type is to love and be loved; the drive for an Earth type is to care and be cared for.

Metal
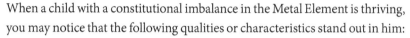

A thriving Metal child

When a child with a constitutional imbalance in the Metal Element is thriving, you may notice that the following qualities or characteristics stand out in him:

- He has an ability to deal with sadness and loss without his spirit becoming compromised.

- He has an appreciation of quality.

- He always does things to the best of his ability.

- He applies himself to his school work and develops a high level of expertise in his areas of interest.

- He has a strong sense of his own worth.

- He is happy in his own company.

A struggling Metal child

When a child with a constitutional imbalance in the Metal Element is struggling, he may have particular difficulties in the following areas:

Sadness and grief

- He is chronically sad.

- He denies any feelings of sadness (he has a 'false sparkle').

- He swings between these two extremes.

- He is nostalgic for the past.

Sense of self

- He has a fragile sense of self-worth.

- He is easily wounded by criticism.

- As a result of this, he tends to cut off from others and distance himself.

- He may be constantly striving, overly perfectionist or overly self-critical.[2]

- His fear of doing things incorrectly stops him from starting things.

- He becomes resigned and cynical.

Other signs of a Metal child

- He may try to impress people with his knowledge (he is really just trying to convince himself of his worth).

- At times, he may have a distinctive white colour to the side of his eyes and around his mouth.

- At times, his voice may have a weeping quality to it, as if he is constantly on the verge of tears.

Ella has a constitutional imbalance in the Metal Element. From a young age, she has shown both a logic and an attention to detail that were beyond her years. Her teachers always praise her for the faultless presentation of her work. She takes so much care over it that sometimes she needs to be encouraged to speed up and not worry so much about missing something out or getting something wrong. Ella's friends always turn to her when they need a voice of calm sense when everybody else is becoming overly emotional. Ella can impress adults with her knowledge and talk very confidently on a wide range of subjects. A small amount of criticism can really floor her, though. Her dad once pointed out a small mistake in her maths and she felt so devastated that it took months of encouragement for her to show him any of her work again. When she gets back from school, she likes to spend some time alone in her room. Being around people all day is quite tiring for her.

Both Fire and Metal children may feel vulnerable in their relationships with others, but for different reasons. A Fire child feels vulnerable to *rejection*, whereas a Metal child feels vulnerable to *criticism*. The key factor for a Fire child is to feel *loved*, whereas the key factor for a Metal type is to feel *appreciated and respected*.

Water
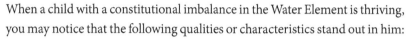
A thriving Water child

When a child with a constitutional imbalance in the Water Element is thriving, you may notice that the following qualities or characteristics stand out in him:

- He is particularly adept at assessing risk.

- He is neither particularly fearful nor reckless.

- He provides others with a great feeling of safety.

- He shows prudence in his approach to rest and activity.

- He is wise (an 'old head on young shoulders').

- He shows great determination and courage.

A struggling Water child

When a child with a constitutional imbalance in the Water Element is struggling, he may have particular difficulties in the following areas:

- He is prone to catastrophic fantasies about the future and is often in a hypervigilant state.

- He rarely ever truly relaxes or switches off.

- He dreads the worst and catastrophises.

- He may become paralysed by fear.

- He is reckless.

- He is chronically agitated and on 'overdrive'.

- He has a lack of drive, willpower or motivation.

Other signs of a Water child

- Others may describe him as 'intense'.

- Others may describe him as 'other-worldly'.

- At times, he may have a blue/black tinge to the side of his eyes and around his mouth.

- At times, his voice may have a groaning quality to it, as if the usual ups and downs of his voice have been flattened.

Jasper has a constitutional imbalance in the Water Element. His mum describes him as a child who has always marched to the beat of his own drum. He has his own strong, internal sense of rhythm and can feel easily stressed when he is asked to do something that goes against this. For example, if he sleeps late and has to rush to get to school he easily ends up having a 'meltdown'. In his friendship group, Jasper is thought of as the one you would want near you in a crisis. He is strong and solid emotionally. However, when he is tired, his parents notice he can easily become quite agitated and fearful. Sometimes, he astounds them with his courage; at other times, he surprises them with how fearful he becomes.

Wood

A thriving Wood child

When a child with a constitutional imbalance in the Wood Element is thriving, you may notice that the following qualities or characteristics stand out in him:

- He is able to be appropriately assertive and handles his angry feelings well.

- He has strong organisational skills.

- He has a strong sense of right and wrong.

- He is capable of great kindness.

- He is able to adapt to changing circumstances.

- He has a strong sense of adventure.

- He is a natural leader.

- He is creative.

A struggling Wood child

When a child with a constitutional imbalance in the Wood Element is struggling, he may have particular difficulties in the following areas:

- He behaves aggressively.

- He is irritable.

- He is moody and petulant.

- He represses his anger and becomes depressed.

- He is overly compliant and lacking in assertion.

- He is impatient.

- He is hyperactive.

- He is inflexible.

Other signs of a Wood child

- At times, his voice is clipped or shouting.

- At times, he has flashes of a green colour around his eyes or mouth.

Amanda has a constitutional imbalance in the Wood Element. She has always known her own mind and had strong views about things. Her friends see her as a leader in their group, and naturally gravitate towards her if a decision needs to be made or somebody needs to take charge. They all think of her as the person they would want to have fight their corner for them. She loves being out and about, having adventures and exploring new things. Her parents know when she is tired because she becomes moody and irritable. Her younger brother calls her 'grumpy and bossy'. She is extremely sensitive to what she perceives as any injustice. If she perceives her brother is getting a better deal than her, she will feel angry and upset.

Both Metal and Wood children may strongly protect their personal boundaries. However, the motivation for each of them is different. A Metal child protects himself because he feels vulnerable to 'attack', in the form of somebody being critical or simply too invasive. A Wood child, on the other hand, may be very boundaried because he has a goal he is trying to reach and does not want anybody to 'get in the way' or frustrate his plans. He is on a mission and does not want to be knocked off course!

Some more clues

Some readers may immediately know which Element relates most to a child in their care. Others may need some more guidance. There are some useful questions to ask yourself which will help you to spot the key Element in a child.

What is the child's default 'tired behaviour'?

Fire: Flat, joyless, sensitive

Earth: Needy, moans, clingy

Metal: Quiet, withdraws, becomes critical of others

Water: Agitated, can't be reassured

Wood: Grumpy, irritable, moody

What makes the child really feel loved?

Fire: Lots of physical affection and warmth; physical presence

Earth: Feeling cared for, understood, thought about and looked after

Metal: Praise and appreciation; sincere and meaningful interaction

Water: Parents and carers tuning in to the child's rhythm

Wood: Having adventures together; being allowed freedom of expression

What motivates the child at school and in life in general?

Fire: The desire to be loved

Earth: The desire to please others

Metal: The desire to achieve excellence

Water: The fear of failure

Wood: The desire to win

What is the child's cry when they are not happy?

Fire: 'I'm bored. Will somebody play with me?'

Earth: 'I don't feel well' or 'I'm worried' or 'I can't cope – will you help me?'

Metal: 'I'm not good enough' or 'I need to be on my own.'

Water: 'I'm scared.'

Wood: 'I'm fed up' or 'It's pointless'.

How does the child approach school work?

Fire: She will work better when work is made to be fun and there are others around.

Earth: She will do twice as much as needed and be overly conscientious.

Metal: She will pay great attention to detail and take a long time over the presentation.

Water: She will show great imagination but may have a tendency to daydream.

Wood: She will rush it so she can get on to the next thing.

What does the child need from a teacher?

Fire: She will respond well to a warm teacher who she likes.

Earth: She will respond well to a teacher who she feels understands and cares for her.

Metal: She will respond well to a teacher who inspires her.

Water: She will respond well to a teacher who allows her to use her imagination.

Wood: She will respond well to an organised teacher who challenges her.

What if I still don't know which Element a child is?

Don't worry! Remember, every child contains each of the Five Elements and sometimes it can be hard to spot the one that is at the root of the child's problems. You might be able to narrow your choice down to two Elements, which is also fine. You can then keep these two Elements in your mind as you observe the child. If you keep paying close attention, you will probably have an 'aha' moment, when you notice something about the child that makes it all fit into place.

So, what now?

Having looked at the different *natures* of each Element type, and how these manifest both when the child is thriving and when she is struggling, we will now turn our attention to the specific kind of *nurture* each child needs.

Endnotes

1 Quoted in E. Slingerland (2015) *Trying Not to Try: The Art of Effortlessness and the Power of Spontaneity* (London: Canongate Books), p. 144.

2 The psychotherapist Julia Samuel calls this tendency to be overly self-critical 'the shitty committee' in our heads: J. Samuel (2020) *This Too Shall Pass: Stories of Change, Crisis and Hopeful Beginnings* (London: Penguin Life), p. 128.

Chapter 5

Nurture: What the Five Element Types Need to Flourish

The big picture

The Five Element character types we have just described are constitutional traits. They are the hand of cards that a child is dealt when he arrives in the world. These are then compounded or modified by the events and circumstances of his life. Any of the five types may become anxious or depressed, but each will do it in his own way.

We will now look at the specific type of nurture that each Element type needs in order to remain free from anxiety or depression. The sorts of things we will talk about are beneficial to every child. However, for some children they may be crucial. Each Element type reacts to his experiences according to his true and unique nature. As the old adage goes, one man's medicine is another's poison.

Essentials for the Fire child

Warmth and intimacy

Almost all parents deeply love their children. Yet so many children grow up feeling unloved. The ability to receive love is a skill. A Fire child may not be as endowed with this skill as another child. There is often a disparity between the way parents express their love, and the ability of the child to receive it. It is as if they are both talking a different language. The love language that a Fire child understands is one that is abundant in warmth and intimacy. Without a good supply of cuddles, eye contact and undiluted attention, the Fire child will struggle to feel loved.

Communication

There are many ways to communicate – not just through speech, but through touch, eye contact and gesture. The Fire child will thrive when there is a lot of healthy, appropriate two-way communication in the family. Communication is like the air that fans the flames of the fire. A Fire child will struggle to thrive in a household where family members live side by side but do their own thing and do not demonstrate much intimacy.

Emotional consistency

The Fire child will struggle if his trusted adults are on an emotional roller coaster and the family home is full of melodrama. Every time there is an emotional 'down', it will trigger his fears of rejection and he will find it hard to remain internally calm and robust. What a Fire child most needs is emotional consistency in those around him.

Security and unconditional love

Of course, every child needs security and to feel that he is unconditionally loved. However, a Fire child will be especially affected by a lack of consistent emotional warmth. His deepest fear is that he is unlovable and that he will be rejected. So it's important that even when he behaves badly or his parents are exhausted and stressed, they still communicate that he is loved. A hastily spoken line in a stress moment of 'I just wish you would go away and leave me alone' might feel very wounding to a sensitive Fire child.

Appreciating sensitivity

A child of any Element type may be sensitive, but Fire children are especially sensitive to behaviour or words that are harsh, unloving or rejecting. He may, for example, feel insecure around a large group of extrovert or straight-talking children who do not appreciate his sensitivities. A Fire child tends to take unkind words or actions very much to heart.

Joy, fun and laughter

A Fire child really needs lots of joy, fun and laughter in his life. He will easily be got down by a sad or joyless emotional atmosphere. A household where everybody is very serious or too busy to stop and have fun will make it hard for a Fire child to thrive. He will benefit from group activities, no matter what they are, as long as they are done in a joyful spirit.

Support with friendships

Friendships and connection are everything to a Fire child. At the same time, this area might be one he finds most challenging. He may need help to right himself after a perceived rejection or need encouragement to socialize if he is feeling especially vulnerable. At other times, a Fire child may need reminding that he cannot always rely on interaction with others to feel joyful. There will be times when he will be on his own and he needs support to manage this.

Essentials for the Earth child
Nurturing parenting

An Earth child needs to feel nurtured, held and understood. He needs to have an abundance of mothering care, whether that comes from his mother or from other adults in his life. The care he receives needs to be particularly well attuned to his needs. If it is not exactly 'right' for him, he will find it hard to receive. He needs to know that his physical and emotional needs will be met in a reliable and timely way.

Stable and harmonious home environment

The Earth Element is often associated with 'the home', and the home environment is particularly important for an Earth child. He needs home to be a place where he feels completely secure. He may also enjoy spending more time at home than other Element types. He needs the household to be harmonious and is a natural diplomat. He may become upset if family members are arguing with each other.

Support to balance his own needs with those of others

An Earth child may feel like he wants to look after everybody else and make sure they are all happy, because he empathises with others' pain so deeply. On the other hand, at times his own needs may feel so overwhelming to him that he has no awareness that others might be struggling too. Whichever is his tendency, he will need guidance to recognise when it is appropriate to focus on his own needs and when he can help others.

Community and tribe

An Earth child will thrive when he feels he is part of a community or tribe. That might be extended family, friendship groups or the local community. It makes him feel supported and connected. He may find it easier to complete a task or do his homework if he is allowed to work together with others, or even have others present. He easily feels overwhelmed by a task if he feels unsupported by others in doing it.

A worry-free environment and help with his worries

An Earth child is prone to worry, overthinking or even obsessive thoughts. If an Earth child grows up with family members who are prone to worry, that will only exacerbate his own tendency to worry. It will also make it hard for him to grow up trusting that his needs will be met and that life will provide for him. When an Earth child does become beset with worry, it is important he has people to whom he can voice his worry. The old adage 'a problem shared is a problem halved' is really true for the Earth child.

Good food and happy eating

The part of the physical body that is associated with the Earth Element in Chinese medicine is the digestive system. It is therefore especially important for an Earth child that he has a good diet and builds up a good relationship with food and eating. In Chapters 15 and 16, we will talk in more detail about food and eating. Suffice it to say here that an Earth child will almost definitely live to eat rather than eat to live, and that food is often a source of emotional and psychological, as well as physical, nourishment for him.

Moderate intellectual stimulation

As I've already discussed, one trait of an Earth child can be the tendency to overthink. Too much intellectual stimulation can exacerbate this trait. Therefore, it is important that an Earth child of school age has a balance between mental and physical activities. If he is feeling overwhelmed and stressed out after a day at school or some tricky homework, the best antidote for him might be to go outside and do something physical.

Both a Fire and an Earth child will benefit from having others around them when they have to get something done. But the reason is different in each case. The Fire child needs others for *stimulation*, whereas the Earth child needs others for *support*.

Essentials for the Metal child

Support to deal with sadness and grief

The emotions associated with the Metal Element are sadness and grief. A Metal child is liable to struggle with these emotions. He needs to be supported to acknowledge sad feelings, express them and then to let them go. If he is given the message that it's 'bad' to feel sad, he will bury these feelings and pretend he is fine. We should not necessarily take the assertion that 'everything is all right' at face value in a Metal child.

Respect and acknowledgement

A Metal child needs particular help to connect with his own sense of worth. He will be especially susceptible to criticism, partly because he may well already be his own worst critic. Instead, what he needs is heartfelt and meaningful praise and acknowledgement for his efforts. He has a deep need for approval. He may feel that whatever he does, it is never good enough. He needs his parents and teachers to remind him that, as Voltaire said, the best is the enemy of the good.

Quality and inspiration

The physical part of the body related to the Metal Element is the respiratory system. Chinese medicine understands that, in order for the Metal Element to thrive, a child needs to breathe in 'the *qi* of the heavens'. What this means in a practical sense is that a Metal child needs people, activities and possessions that will inspire him and connect him to a sense of a higher purpose. One Metal child I know was feeling disengaged from school until he had a science teacher who made the subject come alive and have meaning for him.

Order, clarity and logic

A Metal child needs a home and school environment that is ordered. He needs parents and teachers who are arbiters of right and wrong. If his external world is chaotic, he will struggle to develop a strong internal framework and to feel good about himself. He will also find it difficult if he lives with people who are highly emotional and always let their heart rule their head. Logic and rationality help the Metal child to feel safe and secure.

Help to connect with bodily needs

This tendency to feel secure in the realm of logic and the intellect may mean that he becomes somewhat disconnected from his body. He might look or feel slightly physically awkward and not at home in his body. He may feel uncomfortable with or neglect his basic physical needs, such as eating, exercising or getting enough sleep. He may also find it hard to describe any bodily sensations, such as pain or illness. Touch is one of the best ways to help a Metal child connect with his body, and I will discuss this in more detail in Chapter 9, 'Connection'.

Essentials for the Water child

A feeling of safety

More than anything else, a Water child needs to feel safe. He needs to feel physically and emotionally safe, and that those he loves are safe too. One of the things that most helps him to feel safe is to have adults around him whom he can really trust because they are reliable and solid. A parent who does not turn up when he says he will makes it very difficult for a Water child to feel secure. Similarly, a parent who is filled with anxiety will only increase their Water child's propensity for anxiety and agitation. He needs parents and adults who model to him that the world is not full of danger and potential harms.

Guidance with assessing risk

A Water child may struggle more than another child with risk taking. He may err on the side of being overly cautious, which might prevent him from trying new things and having a full life. On the other hand, he may struggle to know how to keep himself safe. As a teenager, he may be the child whose parents lie awake all night worrying about what risks he is taking. The most important way a parent can help a child like this is to model a balanced approach to risk. As he gets older, conversations are a useful way of encouraging a child to come up with the possible outcomes of an activity *before* he embarks upon it.

Time and space

Just as a river flows at its own pace, a Water child will thrive when he is able to go with his own flow. Of course, a child will always need to learn to follow the constructs of time. However, a Water child will feel stressed when he is made to rush. He also needs psychic space. If he is surrounded by lots of noise and hubbub, he may become tired and irritable. He may have a stronger need than another child for some quiet time on his own, when he can check in with himself and feel peaceful.

Balance of rest and activity

Some Water children are overly driven and, if allowed, would be constantly on the go. Others lack motivation and, if allowed, would spend all day on the sofa. Whichever way he is inclined, a Water child will benefit from encouragement to balance his level of rest and activity. Otherwise, he is in danger of either burning out or becoming a couch potato.

> Both Water and Metal types might need more time on their own than children of other Element types. But they need it for different reasons. The Metal type may feel tired when he has been around a lot of people. The *qi* on the outer surface of his body is not strong so he feels undefended and therefore easily violated. The Water type, on the other hand, feels easily agitated when he is around others. He needs quiet time to regain a sense of inner peace and tranquillity.

Essentials for the Wood child
Support to deal with feelings in the anger family

In many cultures the emotion of anger is thought to be a 'negative' emotion, and this often leads to it being suppressed. In fact, it is a necessary emotion and one that is integral to being a human being. Psychologists understand that many cases of depression are 'frozen rage'. A Wood child may struggle to acknowledge he is angry or to express it in an appropriate way. On the other hand, he may feel constantly frustrated or resentful and behave in an aggressive or destructive way. Ideally, he needs parents and teachers who will model that it is OK to feel angry, but not always to act out from an angry place.

An environment free from conflict and violence

A Wood child may feel particularly stressed when he is in the presence of conflict. It is difficult for a Wood child to tolerate parents who have intense or violent rows. This is because anger is the emotion that resonates with the Wood Element. However, an atmosphere of chronic unspoken resentment or irritation is also one in which it would be difficult for a Wood child to thrive. Even when the anger is not expressed, he will probably sense it unconsciously.

The right balance of freedom versus responsibility

On the one hand, a Wood child needs really clear rules and boundaries in order to feel safe. On the other hand, he needs to be allowed the opportunity to explore, be independent and express his individuality. Just where the sweet spot is between these two will be different for every Wood child. Many Wood children constantly push against boundaries that are set by parents and teachers. Judging what degree of freedom is right for each child at each age is no easy call, but it is one that it is important to try to get right. Too many restrictions and the Wood child will feel stifled and constrained. Too much freedom and a Wood child will feel insecure and unsafe.

Fair and just treatment

A Wood child has a strong sense of fairness and justice, and feels angry when he perceives there has been an injustice, whether against himself or someone else. He will be hypersensitive to any form of favouritism, either from a parent or from a teacher. He feels loved when he is treated fairly, and it may feel to him like a personal violation if parents or teachers are not entirely equitable.

A need to know what's planned

A Wood child is likely to feel secure when he knows what to expect and has prior warning of what is coming next. He likes to have a plan and stick to it. If his parents and teachers are able to take some time to let him know the schedule for the day, it will help him to relax. He may need extra support if things change at the last minute, as flexibility may not be his strength. He is likely to find it difficult to thrive in a household or classroom that is chaotic and when the adults looking after him are disorganized.

Physicality and movement

The Wood Element falls nearer the *yang* end of the *yin/yang* spectrum. This means that a Wood child needs lots of opportunities for movement and physical activity. It may be really hard for him, for example, to sit still at school all day, and he may come home feeling pent-up and irritable. I will discuss exercise and movement more in Chapter 13. A lack of enough movement can be a contributory factor to Wood-type depression.

Elemental nurture checklist
The Fire child

- Is he getting enough overt shows of love and physical affection?

- Is he getting enough time with his parents and other loved ones?

- Is there enough communication within the family, or are family members simply co-existing?

- Is the emotional milieu of the family relatively calm and consistent?

- Are parents and carers aware of the Fire child's sensitivity to harsh words or gestures?

- Is there enough fun, joy and laughter in the Fire child's daily life?

- Is he getting support in navigating his friendships?

The Earth child

- Is she getting the kind of attuned care and motherly nurture she needs?

- Does she have a stable home environment, and enough time in her home?

- Is she being supported to look after her own needs as well as others'?

- Does she feel part of a community or tribe?

- Does she have opportunities to voice her worries to adults who will listen?

- Is she being provided with a good, varied diet?

- Does she have a good balance between intellectual stimulation and other activities?

The Metal child

- Is he given the chance to acknowledge and express any feelings of sadness he may have?

- Is he given lots of heartfelt and meaningful praise and appreciation?

- Does he have activities that give his life meaning and people in his life who inspire him?

- Is his home environment ordered?

- Is he being given clear messages about what is right and wrong?

- Is he being supported to connect with his bodily needs?

The Water child

- Is he surrounded by solid, trustworthy adults who are not themselves chronically anxious?

- Is he being guided to appropriately assess the level of risk in his daily activities?

- Is he given enough time and space to beat to the rhythm of his own drum, or is his life over-scheduled?

- Does he have a good balance of rest and activity in his daily life?

The Wood child

- Is he given support to express feelings in the anger family but not to excessively act out from a place of anger?

- Are his home and school environment relatively free from either expressed or repressed conflict and resentment?

- Is he being given an appropriate level of freedom relative to his nature and his age?

- Are his parents and teachers treating him in a way that is fair and just?

- Is he given forewarning of plans and routines, whenever possible?

- Does he have enough opportunity for movement and exercise?

So, what now?

I hope that you will by now be beginning to understand the Five Element system, and the way it helps us to understand the nature of each individual child and, by extension, the type of care that is particularly important for each and every one. We will now take a deep dive into anxiety and depression, and look at how it manifests differently in different children.

• Chapter 6 •

The Five Types of Anxiety and Depression

The big picture

Before looking at the five types of anxiety and depression, we will first take a more generalised look at each of these two feeling states.

Anxiety

The term 'anxiety' is usually used to describe a *yang*-type feeling, often one that involves a degree of agitation or restlessness. Beyond that, the feeling can have many different flavours. To give but a few examples, it may be that the child feels butterflies in her stomach, or she may have a stream of catastrophic thoughts that she cannot get out of her head; she may have feelings of low self-esteem and, as a result, feel pressure regarding her school work, or she may catastrophise about the future.

Anxiety often shows up as something else

Anxiety in a child often disguises itself as something else. It morphs into a behaviour, a physical symptom or another emotion. For example, the Monday morning stomach ache may be a manifestation of worry about school. It may be that the child does not have either the verbal skills or self-awareness to express how she is feeling.

Sometimes, anxiety shows up as a behaviour. For example, repetitive behaviours, such as opening and closing doors, may arise from anxious-type feelings. The behaviour is the child's way of trying to manage the intense feeling. Sometimes, anxiety shows up as a different emotion. For example, a child may have an outburst of anger when she is asked to do her homework even though her underlying emotion is anxiety about her ability to do it. So, anxiety may show up as:

- a physical symptom

- a behaviour

- another emotion.

Eight-year-old Charlotte was experiencing migraines once or twice a week. They would always come on within an hour or two or coming out of school. On the surface, Charlotte appeared to be a confident and happy child. When I began asking Charlotte about her experience of school, it became obvious that she felt anxious throughout the entire school day and constantly worried that she was not doing well enough in her work. In Charlotte, her anxiety was showing up as migraines. Once she was able to verbalise her anxiety, and with a bit of acupuncture treatment to help reduce it, she no longer suffered from the migraines.

Something else may show up as anxiety

Anxiety can also be a smokescreen. A child may slip into feeling anxious instead of confronting another emotion that she finds too painful. Sometimes, it can be easier to feel anxious than to know ourselves properly. Of course, this all happens unconsciously. For example, a child may talk about feeling 'anxious' but, through dialogue, it becomes apparent that she is seethingly angry or deeply sad. The anxiety has become the means by which she avoids connecting with her anger or sadness.

Fifteen-year-old Christina said she was suffering from high levels of anxiety. As we chatted, I noticed that the emotions Christina was actually expressing were in the anger family. She talked about her irritation with her younger siblings, her fury towards her parents that she was not allowed to stay over at her boyfriend's house and her frustration at studying subjects at school in which she was not interested. Once Christina connected with her anger, and with some acupuncture treatment on her Wood Element, her so-called 'anxiety' became a thing of the past.

Depression

The dictionary defines depression as 'feelings of severe despondency and dejection'.[1] The NHS (UK National Health Service) website says that when someone is depressed, they 'feel persistently sad for weeks or months'.[2] For many, depression has the connotations of a lack of much emotion, a kind of void or emptiness.

However, if you delve deeper into the feeling state of a child who is thought to be depressed, you might find that actually her internal world is characterised by strong and persistent feelings of anger or worry, for example. Or you might find that a teenager who is 'depressed' stays in bed all day not because she feels so sad but because she feels so anxious. The situation is further confused as doctors prescribe what we generally refer to as 'anti-depressant' medications for a wide range of presentations, including anxiety which, in contrast to depression, is characterised by an *excess* of emotion. Anti-depressants are also prescribed for conditions such as eating disorders and self-harm, behaviours that often arise as a result of intense emotions of one kind or another.

From the Chinese medicine perspective, depression can be said to be a *yin*-type feeling because the person tends to go inwards and it is often characterised by a lack of expression. Indeed, expression (which is *yang*) could be said to be the opposite of depression (which is *yin*).

Therefore, as with anxiety, depression can describe many different feeling states. At its root, however, is very often a disconnection from an intense emotion that the child finds too painful to bring to her consciousness. It's as if when disconnected from the energy of that emotion a child is cut off from some of their natural vitality.

● What do we mean by an emotion being painful, and what would cause it to be so? Each emotion has a different impact on a child's *qi*. Some emotions cause movements of *qi* that might lead to a child feeling uncomfortable in his body. It might make him twitchy or restless, for example. A strong emotion may be experienced by a child as being like a tidal wave that engulfs him and induces a loss of control. Or an emotion may be painful because a child expects to be told off or disapproved of if they express it. Alternatively, he may have had an experience when he expressed his fear or worry and was told he should not feel that way. For all these reasons, emotions end up with either positive or negative connotations for a child.

You may be wondering how on earth you are going to understand what is going on in a particular child, bearing in mind that the labels of 'anxiety' and 'depression' cover an almost infinite variety of different emotional states. This is where the Five Element system comes to the fore, enabling us to get to the root of what is really going on emotionally for a particular child.

The five types of anxiety and depression

We discussed in Chapter 4 how the Five Element system is a useful lens through which to view a child's emotional nature. Depending on which Element type a child is, she will have a tendency to experience anxiety and/or depression in a particular way. Her Element type will also mean that particular aspects of life may trigger these uncomfortable feelings in her.

We will now look at the manifestations of anxiety and depression according to each of the Five Elements. Before reading this chapter, you might want to quickly check back to Chapter 4, and remind yourself which of the Five Elements you felt most closely resonated with the child you are concerned about. It might be helpful for you to then look at that Element first in this chapter, and reflect on whether the type of anxiety and/or depression described still seems to fit with that child.

The Fire Element related to anxiety and depression

A child with a constitutional imbalance in the Fire Element will, if he is anxious or depressed, experience and manifest it in a way that resonates with the Fire Element. He may tend to live at one end of the following polarities or the other, or alternate between both ends.

Lack of joy, vitality and spark — Manic, hyper, excessively joyful

Shies away from contact with people — Desperate for contact with people

Wary of intimacy because easily hurt — Wears his heart on his sleeve

Fire anxiety: social anxiety

For the Fire child, his anxiety tends to centre around his friendships and interactions with others. A Fire child may excessively seek out contact with others. Another Fire child may go to great lengths to avoid contact with others. She is caught in a quandary because she needs to feel loved by others to feel OK about herself. At the same time, because she is so dependent on the love of others, she can feel too vulnerable to interact with anybody, for fear of a potential rejection. After interacting with others, she may go over and over what was said to her and what she said, questioning whether she said the right thing and looking for signs that the other person or people liked her.

Fire depression: unloved blues

At the core of a Fire child's depression is a feeling that she is fundamentally unlovable and alone. She will feel flat and, literally, as if her internal Fire has gone out. Her mood may temporarily lift when she is around others but will soon drop again when she is alone.

● You may find it helpful to look back to Chapter 4 at this point, and remind yourself of other characteristics of a Fire child.

Leanne, a fourteen-year-old girl with a constitutional imbalance in Fire, was experiencing high levels of anxiety. Her anxiety focused on her friendships. She had moved to a new school and joined a year group that had already been together for a year. Even though Leanne had quickly become an accepted and much-liked part of a friendship group, she would consistently spend the last couple of hours before bedtime convinced that her new friends did not like her, that she was going to be 'thrown out' of the group and that she had said or done something that day to make herself unpopular. It was this nagging feeling that she was essentially unloved and unlovable that sparked her anxiety. Although this may manifest in milder or more extreme forms, Leanne's is very typical of a Fire-type anxiety.

The core remedy for Fire-type anxiety and depression

Fire-type anxiety and depression is dispelled not through logic, but through love. Relationship and connection need to be prioritised above everything else. Giving warmth, expressing love and spending time with a Fire child is the best medicine.

Please see Chapter 5 in particular for other suggestions for how to help a Fire child feel better.

The areas of life that are particularly important for a Fire child are:

- social media use (see Chapter 12)

- excessive exercise (see Chapter 13)

- sleep (see Chapter 17)

- desire and craving (see Chapter 12)

- overstimulation (see Chapter 12).

The Earth Element related to anxiety and depression

A child with a constitutional imbalance in the Earth Element will, if she is anxious or depressed, experience and manifest it in a way that resonates with the Earth Element. She may tend to live at one end of the following polarities or the other, or alternate between both ends.

Inability to separate from parents and look after self	— Unable to ask for help when necessary
Lack of emotional stability	— Emotionally stolid/phlegmatic
Inability to focus	— Excessive worry and overthinking

Earth anxiety: mental anxiety

At the core of anxiety for an Earth child is the propensity for worry and overthinking. In Chinese medicine, thinking is understood to involve not only the brain but the feelings of the child too. If thinking becomes a purely mental process, it is more likely to become obsessive. The child becomes fixed on the same issue, going over and over it, again and again. This lessens his vitality.

Earth-type 'mental' anxiety may become worse in the lead-up to exams, when the child is required to do more thinking. It also often gets worse at bedtime, and the child may not find it easy to drop off to sleep because of her overactive mind. Ironically, the overthinking can make it harder for her to get down to doing any work, which then perpetuates the worry.

Earth depression: 'it's all too much'

When an Earth child is depressed, her feeling state may be characterised by a sense of being overwhelmed. She complains that she 'can't cope'. Life just simply feels too much for her to manage. She feels weighed down and burdened by the demands that are put upon her. She may also feel that she is not getting enough support. This is often not an external reality, it is just that she cannot truly accept the support she is being given. Therefore, another characteristic of her depression is feeling sorry for herself and as if 'nobody understands' just what she is going through. She becomes rather 'glass half empty' and cannot see what is good in her life.

● You may find it helpful to look back to Chapter 4 at this point, and remind yourself of other characteristics of an Earth child.

Jake, an eleven-year-old with a constitutional Earth imbalance, became very anxious at the thought of separating from his mum. School mornings had become miserable for Jake and his mum, as Jake's anxiety would rise on the journey to school, culminating in him bursting into tears and clinging on to his mum at the school gate. Jake's anxiety also meant he refused all invitations from his friends, and even his grandparents, to sleep over. In all other areas of life, he was very confident. Jake's anxiety was triggered by a fear of how he would cope without his mum being there to look after him. Although this may manifest in milder or more extreme forms, Jake's was a typical Earth-type anxiety.

The core remedy for Earth-type anxiety and depression

When an Earth-type child becomes anxious and/or depressed, a parent may feel worn down by the child's excessive need for sympathy and understanding. They may have a strong urge to tell their child to 'buck up' and stop feeling sorry for herself. However, what most often dispels this child's anxiety and/or depression is being given even more nurture and support. She needs to be allowed to verbalise her worries and other feelings, and for her parent to simply listen and sympathise, rather than offering 'advice' (at least in the first instance). She metaphorically (and perhaps literally) needs an enormous, ongoing hug! It is through feeling that she is truly understood and cared for that she is likely to start feeling unburdened.

Please see Chapter 5 in particular for other suggestions for how to help an Earth child feel better.

The areas of life that are particularly important for an Earth child are:

- diet (see Chapters 15 and 16)

- family (see Chapter 10)

- a balance of physical and mental activities (see Chapter 12)

- sleep (see Chapter 17).

The Metal Element related to anxiety and depression

A child with a constitutional imbalance in the Metal Element, if she is anxious or depressed, experiences and manifests it in a way that resonates with the Metal Element. She may tend to live at one end of the following polarities or the other, or alternate between both ends.

Melancholic and sad — 'False sparkle'

Feeling of worthlessness — Desperate for inspiration and acknowledgement

Inert and unmoved by anything — Fragile and hypersensitive to criticism

Resigned and cynical — Tendency to be in denial of difficulties

Metal anxiety: self-esteem collapse anxiety

For a Metal child, anxiety is usually related to a lack of self-esteem. The child becomes anxious because she feels she is not good enough in some way. She may be anxious about school because she thinks her work will not be good enough, or anxious about playing a team sport in case she lets her team down. The Chinese character for Metal (*jin*) depicts some precious nuggets of gold, covered by layers of soil. The Metal child becomes anxious when she disconnects from those nuggets of gold within herself, and therefore feels herself to be of no value. She may feel it is safer not to try at something, than to try and then (in her own eyes) fail. Her inner critic is often highly developed.

Metal depression: sad and disconnected

A Metal child's depression may arise from overwhelming feelings of sadness. Her nature may mean that she finds it especially difficult to bear sad-type feelings, so she is likely to disconnect from them or get stuck in them. The Chinese character for sadness (*you*) depicts a heart and, below it, a pair of dragging legs. This conveys the idea of a child feeling weighed down by grief or overwhelming sadness.

In our discussion of Fire Element depression, we talked about a child lacking any joyful feelings. This has overlaps with, but is fundamentally different to, the Metal Element feeling of sadness. Fire Element depression is characterised by a flatness and a *lack* of joyful feelings, although in severe cases there can be a more intense element of heartbreak to the feeling. The Metal Element depression is characterised by the *presence* of strong feelings of sadness, loss or grief.

● You may find it helpful to look back to Chapter 4 at this point, and remind yourself of other characteristics of a Metal child.

Aidan, a thirteen-year-old boy with a Metal constitutional imbalance, had been diagnosed with anxiety and depression by his general practitioner and prescribed anti-depressants. For six months he had stopped seeing his friends and only interacted with his family when he really had to. On talking to Aidan, it became apparent that he had an entire committee of voices in his head telling him, 'You don't do that well enough,' or 'You aren't worthy of that person's friendship,' or 'Why do you not have any talents when all your friends have?' It was no wonder he had cut off from his friends and family. Aidan's feelings were triggered by a deep lack of self-worth, which is typical of a Metal-type anxiety and depression.

The core remedy for Metal-type anxiety and depression

The Metal child, above all else, needs acceptance in order to feel better. She needs to know that she is OK just as she is. She is her own worst enemy, and needs to be surrounded by people who are kinder to her than she is to herself. It can really help her if her parents are able to temporarily suspend all expectations and truly accept her even when she is not being high-achieving, well behaved or sociable.

Please see Chapter 5 in particular for other suggestions for how to help a Metal child feel better.

The areas of life that are particularly important for a Metal child are:

- touch (see Chapter 9)

- connection (see Chapter 9)

- appropriate forms of movement and exercise (see Chapter 13)

- breathing (see Chapter 14).

The Water Element related to anxiety and depression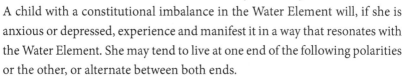

A child with a constitutional imbalance in the Water Element will, if she is anxious or depressed, experience and manifest it in a way that resonates with the Water Element. She may tend to live at one end of the following polarities or the other, or alternate between both ends.

Apathetic — Compulsively pushes self

Paralysed by fear — Agitated and hyperalert

Extremely cautious — Reckless

Water anxiety: existential anxiety

The anxiety experienced by a Water child tends to be pervasive, rather than being focused on one particular aspect of life. She has a natural inclination towards feeling anxious as this is the emotion associated with the Water Element. In this sense, it could be said that Water-type anxiety is a 'true' anxiety, rather than the displacement of another emotion. Having said that, the child may express another emotion (often anger) in the place of anxiety.

A Water child will tend towards being hypervigilant, and experiencing chronic agitation and restlessness. At her core, she lacks a sense of trust that the world is a safe place and that she is safe. Her anxiety tends to get worse when she is tired.

Water depression: a lack of drive

A Water child has more of a tendency to feel anxious than to feel depressed. However, if she does feel depressed, the feeling is often characterised by a lack of drive. She may feel so extremely lethargic that even her normal daily activities just feel like they require too much energy. It may appear as if her will to engage with life and to live is diminished.

● You may find it helpful to look back to Chapter 4 at this point, and remind
yourself of other characteristics of a Water child.

The core remedy for Water-type depression and anxiety

The Water child, above all else, needs reassurance in order to feel better. The
reassurance may come in the form of words. However, she will feel most
reassured by having adults around who are themselves calm and reliable.
She needs to be helped to understand when her fear is unfounded, and to
distinguish between her feelings and reality.

Please see Chapter 5 in particular for other suggestions for how to help
a Water child feel better.

The areas of life that are particularly important for a Water child are:

- balance between rest and activity (see Chapter 12)

- the emotional environment of the family (see Chapter 10)

- sleep (see Chapter 17)

- exercise (see Chapter 13).

Leah, an eight-year-old girl with a Water constitutional imbalance, had
been feeling increasingly anxious over the last year. She often woke at 5
a.m. and within minutes she would be catastrophising about all the things
that might go wrong that day.[1] Leah was also very anxious about going
to new places or trying a new activity. Even when she was at home, she
almost always felt a degree of agitation. Her mother felt that her fears
were impacting on her ability to live a full life. Although this may manifest
in milder or more extreme forms, Leah's was a typical Water-type anxiety.

The Wood Element related to anxiety and depression

A child with a constitutional imbalance in the Wood Element will, if she is
anxious or depressed, experience and manifest those feelings in a way that
resonates with the Wood Element. She may tend to live at one end of the
polarities or the other, or alternate between both ends.

---

1   The *qi* of the Water Element is at its lowest between 5 a.m. and 7 a.m., so symptoms of an
imbalance in this Element may become worse at this time of day.

Feels hopeless, gloomy and moody — Overtly or covertly angry

Overly compliant and lacking in — Defiant
assertiveness

Unable to make decisions, — Controlling and inflexible
lacking in direction

Wood anxiety: stress and pressure anxiety

The Wood child's anxiety is a response to the stress of daily life. At its heart, it is often related to feeling 'stressed out' by everything that has to be done, and the child's daily schedule or to-do list. She may try to quell her anxiety by excessively making plans. Her anxiety is often better during holidays when the pressure is off. The child may say that she feels 'tense'. There is a sense that she has tensed up in order to be able to get through what is expected of her.

Wood depression: 'what's the point?' depression

The Wood child's depression is characterised by negative thoughts, usually along the lines of 'what's the point?' or 'the future is hopeless'. These thoughts often arise because of inward-turned anger. The child may be fuming or not express anger, or even know that she is angry. Her experience is one of hopelessness. If she does have an outburst of anger, she often feels better for it.

Wood-type anxiety and depression tend to get worse premenstrually in girls.

● You may find it helpful to look back to Chapter 4 at this point, and remind yourself of other characteristics of a Wood child.

The core remedy for Wood-type depression and anxiety

In order to quell her anxiety, a Wood child needs to feel less pressured. This usually means reducing her daily commitments and paring back her routine. In order to feel less depressed, a Wood child also needs to be supported in recognising that she has feelings in the anger family (e.g. irritability, frustration) and then to find a way of expressing them that is not destructive towards others. Aristotle wrote, 'It is easy to fly into a passion – anybody can do that – but to be angry with the right person to the right extent and at the right time and with the right object and in the right way – that is not easy, and it is not everybody who can do it.' His words are especially relevant for a child with a Wood constitutional imbalance.

Please see Chapter 5 in particular for other suggestions for how to help a Wood child feel better.

The areas of life that are particularly important for a Wood child are:

- emotions (see Chapter 8)

- day-to-day life (see Chapter 12)

- exercise (see Chapter 13).

Jeeva, a thirteen-year-old girl with a Wood constitutional imbalance, had been experiencing an increasingly low mood over the past year or so. She said that she felt as if life was a bit pointless, and she just couldn't be bothered with anything. Her parents experienced her as moody and irritable. As Jeeva opened up, she began expressing her anger at having to move from the city to the country and leave her friends behind. She also thought that the many rules at her new school were over the top and served no purpose. Jeeva's low mood was a typical Wood-type depression, characterised by inward-turned anger. As she began to express her angry feelings, her mood lifted.

Table 6.1 The five types of anxiety and depression

	FIRE	EARTH	METAL	WATER	WOOD
Anxiety	Social	Mental	Self-esteem collapse	Existential	Stress and pressure
Depression	Unloved blues	It's all too much	Sad and disconnected	Lack of drive	What's the point?

So, what now?

We have now seen the many nuanced and varied ways in which anxiety and depression can manifest in children of different elemental types. Some cases will be fairly straightforward and, from what you have read, you will be feeling confident that the child you have in mind is a Wood child and the way she manifests her anxiety is typical of a Wood-type anxiety.

In other cases, you may feel that things are not quite so clear. You feel that the child in mind is a Fire child but her anxiety seems to resonate more with the description of an Earth child. Or that her anxiety is a Metal-type anxiety and her depression is more like that of a Water-type depression. That's OK! Human beings are complicated and rarely show up just as the books say. If two or more Elements keep coming to mind for one particular child, you can look at the advice that pertains in particular to both those two Elements.

We are now going to go a step further in terms of our understanding of anxiety and depression. The Five Element understanding gives us a crucial overview. However, under the umbrella of each Element, there are further variations related to the Vital Substances (which we discussed in Chapter 2) and the organs associated with each Element.

Endnotes

1   Lexico (n.d.) 'Depression'. www.lexico.com/definition/depression
2   www.nhs.uk/conditions/clinical-depression

• Chapter 7 •

The *Yin/Yang* of Anxiety and Depression

The big picture

In the previous chapter, we looked at anxiety and depression through the lens of the Five Elements. We are now going to look at them through the lens of the Vital Substances. You might want to check back to Chapter 2 to remind yourself of their nature before reading further. Having established which Element is struggling the most in a child, the next step is to ascertain which of her Vital Substances are out of kilter in some way. This will provide a further level of detail, and help you to hone the lifestyle advice relevant to that child.

A *yin/yang* perspective of anxiety and depression

In broad terms, anxiety is a *yang* emotion or state. It is characterised by an agitation and restlessness. In contrast, depression is a *yin* feeling state. It is characterised by stillness.

Anxiety and depression are often referred to almost as if they are two aspects of a whole. It is indeed the case that a child who feels anxious will, at times, feel low. It is also the case, as mentioned before, that a child who feels low may do so because he has lots of anxious feelings which are 'stagnant'.

We discussed in Chapter 1 how *yin* and *yang* are two poles of a duality, completely interdependent and in constant tension with one another. If we understand anxiety as *yang* and depression as *yin*, the same can be said for these two feeling states. They are interconnected and co-exist, and at any time one or other may predominate. A child may have a tendency to stay at the more *yang* anxious end of the spectrum, or the more *yin* depressed end of the spectrum. He may flip between the two. He may also appear on the surface to be more *yin* and depressed, but this may be a cover for a more *yang*, anxious state.

If a child's emotional state tends to be more *yang* in nature, then what the child needs to feel better is more *yin* aspects to his daily life. For example, a highly agitated child will benefit from rest, rhythm, peace and quiet and a low-stimulation lifestyle. If, on the other hand, his emotional state tends to be more *yin* in nature, then what he needs is more *yang* aspects to his life. For example, he may benefit from more movement and exercise, appropriate stimulating activities and encouragement to express his emotions.

Disharmonies of the Vital Substances in anxiety and depression

Having outlined the key Chinese medicine ideas related to anxiety and depression, we will now look at particular patterns of disharmony of the Vital Substances.

Deficient patterns

Deficient pathologies are those where one of the Vital Substances is *lacking* or where there is an underactivity of one of the functions of an organ or substance. The remedy is always to focus on *nourishing, strengthening* or *building* whichever substance is deficient.

Blood deficiency: causing the *shen* to be slightly disturbed or deficient

We explored the Chinese medicine concept of *blood* in Chapter 2. *Blood* is of paramount importance for the mental/emotional health of a child because of its function of 'housing' the *shen*. If the *shen* is not housed, there will inevitably be some mental/emotional dysfunction. *Blood* deficiency is most commonly seen in relation to an imbalance in the Fire Element and/or the Wood Element. The main reasons *blood* becomes deficient in a child are:

- poor diet (see Chapters 15 and 16)

- excessive exercise (see Chapter 13)

- excessive studying (see Chapter 12)

- the onset of menstruation in girls.

MENTAL/EMOTIONAL SYMPTOMS

- Mild anxious feelings
- Socially anxious
- Feels low and lacking in spark
- Easily tearful
- Easily hurt
- Takes time to get off to sleep or wakes during the night

ACCOMPANYING PHYSICAL SYMPTOMS

- A feeling of agitation in the chest
- Difficulty concentrating for long periods of time
- Light-headed when stands up
- Poor short-term memory
- Tendency to easily startle
- Tired

SOME OUTWARD SIGNS YOU MIGHT NOTICE

- Her complexion is a dull-pale colour
- Her nails are brittle or ridged

BETTER FOR:

- rest
- lying down
- breaks from study and stress
- *blood*-nourishing diet (see Chapter 16).

WORSE FOR:

- excessive study

- over-exercise

- onset of menstruation in girls

- after a heavy period in girls.

If the child you have in mind is *blood* deficient, ask yourself the following questions:

- Is she eating enough *blood*-nourishing foods? (See Chapter 16)

- Is she 'over'-exercising, relative to her age and constitution? (See Chapter 13)

- Is she doing too many mental/head-based activities? (See Chapter 12)

- How many hours of sleep is she getting each night? (See Chapter 17)

- Is she spending a long time on social media and on an emotional roller coaster as a result of it? (See Chapter 12)

Once you have identified the cause or causes of a child's *blood* deficiency, and implemented the necessary lifestyle changes, you may notice an improvement in symptoms within approximately a month. However, depending on the child and her constitution, it may take a few more months before the *blood* deficiency is completely 'cured', or it may be something that needs ongoing attention (especially in menstruating girls).

BLOOD DEFICIENCY ANXIETY

Ten-year-old Lucy (whose constitutional imbalance was in the Fire Element) had begun to feel low and slightly anxious. She found it did not take much for her to get into a really worried state, and she lacked her usual vitality and spark. Through chatting to Lucy, we traced the onset of her change in mood to a couple of months after she had become vegan. Lucy's vegan diet consisted of pasta and not much else. She was barely eating anything that helped to build her *blood* and keep it strong. She was so fed up with feeling low and anxious that she decided to include some ethically sourced and organic fish and meat into her diet four or five times a week, as well as to increase her range of vegetables and pulses. Within three months, Lucy was feeling back to her old self.

Yin deficiency: causing the shen to be deficient or disturbed

We explored the concept of *yin* way back in Chapter 1. *Yin* has a calming, grounding effect on the emotions. It enables a child to have a stillness of mind. It needs to be strong to counterbalance *yang*, in order to prevent a child from feeling excessively agitated. The *yin* of any Element may become deficient, but in children and teenagers the Water and Fire Elements are commonly affected. The most common reasons for a child to become *yin* deficient are:

- constitutional

- over-scheduled lifestyle (see Chapter 12)

- excessive exercise (see Chapter 13)

- excessive scrutiny (see Chapter 10).

MENTAL/EMOTIONAL SYMPTOMS

- Anxious feelings which are worse in the evening and when tired

- A feeling of unease

- Wakes early in the morning, feeling anxious

- Tendency to easily become hyperactive when anxious

- Seeks constant reassurance that they are safe

- May lash out in anger when anxious

ACCOMPANYING PHYSICAL SYMPTOMS

- Feels hot or sweats at night

- May have urgency of bowels and/or bladder when anxious

- Tendency to bed-wetting

- Struggles to relax or be still

SOME OUTWARD SIGNS YOU MIGHT NOTICE

- Her face becomes easily flushed, especially in the afternoon and evenings

- Her body is rarely completely still

BETTER FOR:

- rest

- slower pace of life.

WORSE FOR:

- overstimulation

- excessive exercise

- excessive pressure.

If the child you have in mind is *yin* deficient, ask yourself the following questions:

- What is her daily schedule like? Does it contain a good balance of activity relative to rest? (See Chapter 12)

- Is her level of activity appropriate considering her age and constitution? (See Chapter 13)

- How many hours of sleep is she getting per night? (See Chapter 17)

Once you have identified the cause or causes of a child's *yin* deficiency, and implemented the necessary changes to her lifestyle, you will start noticing some improvement in the child's symptoms within approximately three months. However, *yin* deficiency can take many more months to be completely 'cured'. In some children, especially those with a constitutional deficiency of *yin*, it may be something that needs ongoing attention.

YIN DEFICIENCY ANXIETY

Fourteen-year-old Greg began feeling anxious about a year after he moved to secondary school. He found he could never fully relax and had even had a full-on panic attack a couple of times. He loved his new school, but his schedule was relentless. He got up at 6 a.m. every day, got to school at 7.30 a.m. and didn't get back home until 6.30 p.m. He then spent a couple of hours doing homework, and a few times a week had a sporting activity in the evening too. Greg had been born prematurely, and consequently his physical constitution was slightly weak. He was growing very fast at this age. He simply could not handle this kind of schedule and a growth spurt at the same time. He was digging into his reserves of *yin* in order to get through the day. It was not easy to find ways of reducing Greg's schedule, particularly because he loved all of it! However, Greg stopped his evening sports, made sure he got to bed an hour earlier each night, and left one day free every weekend to completely wind down. These changes helped to some degree and once Greg had stopped growing quite so fast, things got better still.

Qi deficiency: causing the *shen* to be deficient

In Chapter 2, we discussed how the concept of *qi* lies at the very heart of Chinese medicine. *Qi* is the 'vital force' that fuels every cell in a child's body. The vast majority of children will, at some point or another, have some degree of *qi* deficiency. For some children, it is an almost constant state, due to a combination of constitution and lifestyle.

Qi deficiency can affect the organs associated with any Element, but most commonly affects the Earth, Water and Metal Elements. However, *qi* deficiency only ever tends to cause relatively mild mental/emotional symptoms. The most common reasons a child becomes *qi* deficient are:

- his day-to-day life does not allow for enough downtime and rest

- he is overstimulated

- he does not have a sufficiently nourishing diet

- he does too much exercise

- he does not get enough sleep.

MENTAL/EMOTIONAL SYMPTOMS

- Tendency to worrying and overthinking

- Over-attentive to surroundings and other people

- Tends towards obsessive thinking

ACCOMPANYING PHYSICAL SYMPTOMS

- Easily tired

- Lacks vitality

- Loose stools

- Poor appetite

- Breathlessness on exertion

SOME OUTWARD SIGNS YOU MIGHT NOTICE

- The child looks pale

BETTER FOR:

- rest

- nourishing food

- reduced activity and stimulation.

WORSE FOR:

- lack of sleep

- poor diet

- too much exercise

- excessive studying.

If the child you have in mind is *qi* deficient, ask yourself the following questions:

- Does he have a good balance of rest and activity in his daily life? (See Chapter 12)

- Is he getting enough sleep for his age and constitution? (See Chapter 17)

- Does he have an adequately nourishing diet? (See Chapters 15 and 16)

- Is he doing too much exercise relative to his age and constitution? (See Chapter 13)

Once you have identified the cause or causes of a child's *qi* deficiency, and implemented the necessary changes to his lifestyle, you will be likely to start noticing some improvement within a week or two. *Qi* deficiency is relatively quick and easy to 'cure', compared with the other deficiency patterns.

Full patterns

Full patterns are those where there is an *excess* of something in the child's body, either because the body has been 'invaded' by an external pathogenic factor (which Western medicine would usually call bacteria or viruses) or some bodily function has become overactive. A full pattern may be an accumulation of a Vital Substance or a blockage of some kind.

Qi stagnation: causing the *shen* to be disturbed

In the Classics of Chinese medicine, stagnation was understood to be almost synonymous with depression. Although, in reality, depression can come from other causes, stagnation of *qi* is one of the most commonly seen. In the vast majority of cases it is related to the Wood Element and, specifically, the Liver organ. Any emotion, when it becomes blocked or stuck, can lead to stagnation of *qi*, although emotions in the anger family are most commonly at the root of it. When a child is depressed, we need to be a detective and find out which emotion has become blocked. Often, once this emotion is freed up, the feeling of depression is relieved. The most common causes of *qi* stagnation are:

- blocked, repressed or unexpressed emotions

- lack of movement and activity

- an over-scheduled lifestyle

- too much constraint and not enough freedom.

MENTAL/EMOTIONAL SYMPTOMS

- Tendency to feel low and hopeless

- Grumpy, moody and irritable

- Intermittently flares with anger

- Feels uptight and tense

- Lacks dreams, plans, aspirations and a vision of the future

- Feels worse in the morning, when he has not moved or when frustrated

- Worse premenstrually in girls

ACCOMPANYING PHYSICAL SYMPTOMS

- Headaches

- Tense neck and shoulders

- Tight body

- Abdominal cramps and/or distention

- Alternating constipation and diarrhoea

- Belching and flatulence

- Frequent yawning

- Difficulty in breathing, with a tight chest

SOME OUTWARD SIGNS YOU MIGHT NOTICE

- The child's body looks tense

- Her voice may be loud or shouting

BETTER FOR:

- movement

- expressing anger and frustration

- reducing schedule.

WORSE FOR:

- lack of movement and exercise

- repressing angry feelings

- being over-scheduled

- a lack of freedom and independence

- premenstrually in girls.

In some children, *qi* stagnation affects the head in particular. As well as depression, this can also cause:

- inflexible thinking

- difficulty in dealing with any kind of change or an altered routine

- limited emotional expression

- in severe cases, a desire to bang his head repeatedly against something hard

- hypersensitivity to noise.

Appendix 2 outlines some massages that are effective at treating this pattern of imbalance.

If the child you have in mind has *qi* stagnation, ask yourself the following questions:

- Is he repressing an emotion? If so, which emotion? (See Chapter 8)

- Does his daily life contain enough movement and activity? (See Chapter 13)

- Is there enough downtime in his schedule? (See Chapter 12)

- Is he being given the space to express his individuality and test his independence?

Once you have identified the cause or causes of a child's *qi* stagnation, and implemented the necessary changes to his lifestyle, you will be likely to start noticing some improvement within a week or two. Once the *qi* is unblocked, the mental/emotional state of the child can change very quickly. However, exercise may only provide a temporary solution if there is a repressed emotion at the root of the problem.

QI STAGNATION DEPRESSION

Sixteen-year-old Max had been feeling so depressed he was struggling to get out of bed in the mornings and go to school. He felt everything was just pointless and hopeless. At the weekends, he barely made it out of bed and slept a lot of the time, although he never felt better for the sleep. His low mood had begun quite suddenly. It seemed to tie in with his best friend getting a girlfriend, and no longer being around to hang out with him.

Max said he understood that his friend would want to spend all his time with his new girlfriend. Even though in his head he understood this, at a feeling level, he was furious. The anger only rose to the surface when he had an argument with his friend, who'd said he was not available to go to a football match together as they had always done. Once he had expressed his anger, he immediately began to feel a lot better. It meant his *qi* began flowing more smoothly and unblocked his depressed feeling.

Damp-phlegm: causing the *shen* to be clouded

Damp-phlegm is essentially a build-up of fluids in the body. It tends to appear gradually, over weeks and months. Some children will have a constitutional tendency to this pattern. It can appear in a child with any elemental constitutional imbalance, but is most common in an Earth child. The most common causes of *damp-phlegm* are:

- a diet of *damp-phlegm*-forming foods (see Chapter 16)

- a lack of exercise (see Chapter 13).

MENTAL/EMOTIONAL SYMPTOMS

- Feels low, unmotivated and 'heavy'

- Wants to sleep all the time

- Does not want to move

- Struggles to think clearly

- Feels disconnected from others

ACCOMPANYING PHYSICAL SYMPTOMS

- Heavy, stuffy feeling in chest

- Muzzy, 'cotton wool' head

- Lack of thirst

- Catarrh

SOME OUTWARD SIGNS YOU MIGHT NOTICE

- The child has a tendency to greasy skin

- She has a puffy face

- She has a tendency to being overweight

BETTER FOR:

- movement and activity.

WORSE FOR:

- first thing in the morning

- lack of movement

- too much dairy, oily and greasy food.

If the child you have in mind has the *damp-phlegm* pattern, ask yourself the following questions:

- Does his diet contain a lot of dairy, sugar, fatty and/or oily foods? (See Chapter 16)

- Does he have enough movement and activity in his daily life? (See Chapter 13)

If the child is able to change his diet, his low feelings may begin to lift quite quickly. Depending on the constitution of the child, he may begin to feel better within a couple of weeks. This pattern commonly goes hand in hand with an underlying *qi* deficiency. So once the signs of *damp-phlegm* have receded, it is useful to then address the causes of the *qi* deficiency.

Heat: causing the *shen* to be disturbed

Heat can be understood as an imbalance of *yin/yang*, where *yang* has become excessive, or Fire has begun burning out of control. *Heat* tends to rise, and in so doing reaches the Heart, where the *shen* is housed. This tends to bring about an agitating effect. *Heat* can arise purely as a result of *yin* being deficient, but also because something in the child's life is stimulating the production of *heat* in the body. *Heat* that causes mental/emotional problems most commonly affects the Fire and/or Wood Elements, both of which are *yang* in nature. The most common causes of *heat* in a child are:

- intense emotions

- emotional melodrama

- alcohol and recreational drugs

- a diet containing a lot of spicy food

- constitutional.

MENTAL/EMOTIONAL SYMPTOMS

- Severe anxiety

- Panic attacks

- Feels as if heart is pounding in chest

- Extreme agitation

- Extreme sleep disturbance – awake for long periods during the night

- Sleep is disturbed by dreams

ACCOMPANYING PHYSICAL SYMPTOM

- Feels very thirsty

SOME OUTWARD SIGNS YOU MAY NOTICE

- Red face and eyes
- Extreme physical restlessness

BETTER FOR:

- emotional stability
- a cooling diet
- cutting out recreational drugs and alcohol.

WORSE FOR:

- stress
- intense emotions or emotional melodrama
- lack of exercise
- spicy foods
- alcohol and recreational drugs.

If the child you have in mind has a *heat* pattern, ask yourself the following questions:

- What in the child's life is causing her to have intense, strong emotions? (See Chapter 8)
- Is she using recreational drugs and/or alcohol?
- Does her diet contain a lot of spicy food? (See Chapter 16)

EXCESS *HEAT* ANXIETY

Nine-year-old Shona had been experiencing severe anxiety for the last six months. The onset of her anxiety coincided almost exactly with the time her parents had announced they were going to separate. Due to financial constraints, the family still lived together and her parents were having heated rows almost every evening. Shona was a sensitive Fire child and she was deeply upset both by the fact her parents were separating and by the rows. Unfortunately, her parents continued to row but the following steps helped to reduce Shona's level of anxiety, until her father eventually moved out and the rows stopped.

- Shona and her mum went for a walk in nature every day after school, come rain or shine.

- Shona's mum worked extra hard to make sure Shona ate a 'neutral' diet, avoiding spicy foods, additives or too much sugar (see Chapter 16).

- Shona did some breathing exercises every morning and evening (see Chapter 14).

- Shona's mum did *'shen* calming' massage techniques (see Appendix 1) every night.

Combined patterns

Sometimes, a child will clearly suffer from one of the patterns of imbalance described in this chapter. At other times, the child will have a mix of two or more patterns. This means he will show signs and symptoms of both. Any pattern of imbalance may combine with another. However, the following combinations are common:

- *Yin* deficiency and *heat*

- *Qi* and *blood* deficiency

- *Qi* deficiency and *damp-phlegm*

- *Blood* deficiency and *qi* stagnation

If a child has more than one pattern of imbalance, then it is helpful to focus first on the one that predominates.

Relating patterns of disharmony to severity of symptoms

The following diagrams illustrate how each of the patterns of disharmony we have discussed in this chapter are likely to cause different severities of anxiety and depression.

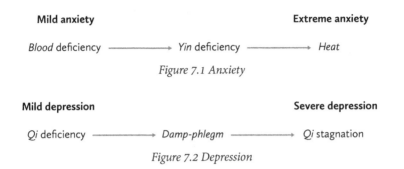

Mild anxiety   **Extreme anxiety**

Blood deficiency ⟶ *Yin* deficiency ⟶ *Heat*

Figure 7.1 Anxiety

Mild depression   **Severe depression**

Qi deficiency ⟶ *Damp-phlegm* ⟶ *Qi* stagnation

Figure 7.2 Depression

So, what now?

By now, you will have some understanding of how Chinese medicine views anxiety and depression, from both a Five Element and a Vital Substances perspective. If you are reading this book with a particular child in mind, you probably have some thoughts about which Element and other patterns of imbalance might be applicable to them.

In Part 2, you will learn how all the key areas of a child's life can impact on his mental/emotional health and, crucially, how you can modify them in order to optimise his well-being, lift his mood and quell his anxiety.

Part 2

HELPING

. . . .

Chapter 8

Emotions

The big picture

Emotions lie at the core of what makes us human. Even if we are not always aware of them, we experience them from the moment we are born until the day we die. The nature of our emotions and the way we manage them arguably make more of a difference to the quality of our lives than any other single factor.

There is so much of life that we have no control over, yet we can influence our emotional response to what happens. However, our society does little to help children learn the skill of recognising and managing emotions.

Children today are growing up in the era of social media, where almost the only emotion that is ever put on display is happiness. Consequently, many children and teens think there is something wrong with feeling any other emotion, such as anger or sadness. Furthermore, emotions can be uncomfortable. We are motivated so strongly in the 21st century by comfort, ease and instant gratification. Sitting with 'difficult' emotions therefore goes against the grain.

For these reasons, children often try to get rid of or run away from feelings of anger, sadness or fear. In the 21st century, it takes commitment not to be distracted from our emotions. It is all too easy to pick up a phone and start scrolling when we sense the rumblings of agitation or distress within us. The more a child avoids an emotion, the more power it begins to have over him. As Proust said in *A la Recherche du Temps Perdu*, 'We are healed of our suffering only by experiencing it to the full.' The aim is to metabolise emotions rather than suppress them or resist them.

The way to prevent emotions becoming a cause of mental/emotional dysfunction, therefore, is to make friends with them.

The Chinese medicine view of emotions

Chinese medicine has always understood emotions to be a potential cause of imbalance. An early Chinese medical text called the *San Yin Fang* (1174) explained that emotions in themselves are not problematic. But they become so when they are intense, when they are prolonged or when they are repressed or unresolved. This is when emotions can become detrimental to a child's mental/emotional state.

Emotions are movements of *qi*

Emotions are a response of the *shen* to stimuli from the outside world. Chinese medicine views emotions as physiological events, or as strong movements of *qi* within the body. These derangements of *qi* occur simultaneously at a physical and an emotional level.

To take fear as an example, a child may feel palpitations, have a sudden need to empty her bowels or start shivering. There is usually a physical response to the emotion, as well as a feeling response. This is why Chinese medicine is often described as being able to treat the mind and body. In fact, it does not really distinguish between mind and body. Human beings are simply *qi* and anything (e.g. an emotion) that affects *qi* will therefore affect the whole person.

Each emotion moves *qi* in a particular way

We know that feeling fearful is a very different experience to feeling sad. We know that if we erupt with fury, we will feel very different than if we sob with sadness. Just as a breeze will move through trees in a very different fashion than would a hurricane, each emotion travels through the body in its own fashion and leaves a different footprint. Later on in this chapter, we will delve deeper into the individual effects of each emotion.

When we are caring for a child and trying to understand more about his emotional world, having a sense of the different energetic quality of each emotion can be very helpful. Observing outward signs of inner emotions is often a more reliable way of understanding what is going on in a child than purely listening to what she says.

Intense, prolonged or repressed emotions disturb the balance of *qi* in the child

So, how do emotions become a cause of mental/emotional dysfunction? They do this by altering the flow of *qi* within the child. They cause internal disharmony. An intense, prolonged or repressed emotion is the metaphorical equivalent of a strong gale, a tornado or a hurricane. It will leave some disruption in its wake. It will make it very difficult for the child to get back to a balanced state, so she is left with disordered *qi*. The exact way in which the *qi* becomes disordered depends on the particular emotion or emotions involved.

Disordered *qi* leads to disordered emotions

However, this is not a one-way street. The disruption in the child's *qi* that the emotion leaves behind then leads to the feeling and expression of emotions becoming more disrupted.

If a child's *qi* is not flowing smoothly, she will be prone to getting 'stuck' in an emotion or feeling an emotion very intensely. This of course then leads to more disrupted *qi* flow. So a vicious circle has been created, from which it can be hard for the child to escape.

And how does this lead to anxiety and/or depression?

Anxiety and depression are in themselves an expression of *qi* that has become disordered. They rarely develop after low-level or short-term *qi* disruption. However, if a child feels particular emotions over a period of time, or suffers a severe one-off trauma, her *qi* may become so disordered that she cannot find her way back to feeling 'herself'. It is as if her body becomes so accustomed to working in a dysfunctional way that this becomes her new normal. Her *qi* is then characterised by dysfunction.

Another way of saying this is that the child's spirit has become affected. She has crossed the line between an emotional turbulence that is part and parcel of life, and one that has begun to compromise her quality of life.

So, to summarise:

- Intense, prolonged or repressed emotions disturb the balance of *qi* in a child.

- An imbalanced flow of *qi* then leads to disordered emotions.

- Disordered emotions then disturb the flow of *qi* even more.

- At some point, the child cannot find her way back to a 'normal' and healthy *qi* state.

- At this point, anxiety and/or depression may set in.

Figure 8.1 shows how disordered emotions may eventually lead to anxiety and/or depression.

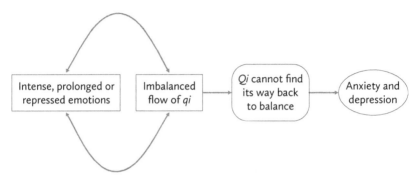

Figure 8.1 How disordered emotions lead to anxiety and/or depression

The seven emotions

One of the Chinese medical classics, the *Simple Questions*, describes in great detail the different emotions and the particular effect they may have upon a person's *qi*. In the West, we tend to have rather fixed ideas about whether a particular emotion is positive or negative. However, emotions are not in themselves inherently good or bad. They are simply responses to the world around us and to our experiences. Emotions can be understood as movements of *qi*, each one having its own particular quality. A surge of anger, for example, feels very different to wallowing in sadness.

We will now look at the nature of each emotion and the effect it might have on a child's *qi*.

Joy

The emotion of joy resonates with the Fire Element. Excessive joy makes the *qi* 'loose', by which we mean it can create agitation and a loss of control. It is a *yang* emotion. This is very easily seen in children after a birthday party, for example, when joy tips over into tears and unhappiness. This is usually temporary and not something to be concerned about.

However, a long-term lack of joy is commonly both a symptom and a cause of imbalance. If a child lacks warm relationships, fun and happiness, or if she is constitutionally a Fire type, the *qi* of her Fire Element is likely to lack vibrancy and strength. The less vibrant and strong the *qi* of the Fire Element, the harder it is for the child to feel joyful.

Signs of a lack of joy

- Lack of spontaneous laughter, cheer, *joie de vivre* and vitality
- Any joy or laughter quickly subsides once the stimulus for it is over
- Voice sounds flat

Sadness

The emotion of sadness resonates with both the Fire and the Metal Elements. Sadness overlaps with lack of joy but has more intensity. It might manifest as a kind of melancholy which is akin to a feeling of heartbreak or devastation.

Sadness tends to suppress or deplete the *qi* of both these Elements. It is a *yin* emotion. Any loss a child experiences may cause her to experience sadness – moving away from a much-loved friend, the death of a grandparent, or the break-up of her parents' relationship, for example.

Signs of sadness

These are similar to those listed under 'Signs of a lack of joy' but also:

- Feels deeply hurt

Worry

The emotion of worry resonates with the Earth Element. Its effect on a child's *qi* is to cause it to become 'knotted'. If a child's *qi* is knotted, then her thoughts become stuck and go around and around. In extreme cases, her thoughts may even become obsessive. It becomes impossible for her to translate thought into action. Of course, the more knotted her *qi* becomes, the more prone to worry and preoccupation she is. An Earth-type child may be particularly prone to this, but it's common to see it in children of any Element type around exam time, for example.

Signs of worry

- Tendency to ruminate and become preoccupied
- Worries are worst in the evening and at bedtime
- Struggles to turn thoughts into actions
- Worries may be accompanied by tummy aches or upset bowels
- A singing tone or a strong lilt to the voice

Grief

Grief may sound much the same as sadness. However, the Chinese differentiate between these two emotions. As we saw, sadness tends to deplete the *qi* of both the Fire and Metal Elements. Grief, however, particularly resonates with the Metal Element and tends to have a heavy, dragging or oppressive effect on a child's *qi*. It is an intensely *yin* emotion. In this context the word 'grief' does not only mean emotions evoked by the loss of a loved one – grief can arise for many different reasons. A child might feel a sense of loss on leaving a school, or even of a particular time in her childhood, or miss a friend who moves away.

It is common to hear parents say that their child does not seem to be affected by a loss of some kind. However, grief is not always easy to spot. When faced with great loss, a child often withdraws as a sort of protection mechanism. She may feel that every interaction may lead to her *qi* 'escaping' and she needs to hide herself away to protect what remains. Sometimes this means she comes across as emotionally cold or inert, but this is only because she is internally busy trying not to become overwhelmed by her feelings.

Signs of grief

- A tendency to withdraw
- Chest is sunken and shoulders are hunched over
- Voice has a weeping tone to it (as if the child is constantly on the verge of tears)

Fear

The emotion of fear resonates with the Water Element. Fear is said to make the *qi* of the Water Element 'descend'. It is a *yin* emotion. In children, there are often obvious physical effects of *qi* descending, such as bed-wetting.

A one-off fright, when it is not so severe as to really shock the child, is unlikely to be problematic in the long term. However, a state of ongoing fear or anxiety is much more deleterious to the balance of a child's *qi*. On a mental/emotional level, chronic fear tends to lead to agitation. It means that the child is always on edge, stuck in what is often termed a 'fight or flight' state. She may be constantly looking for the next threat and create catastrophic fantasies, for example, of her parents dying. A child who is stuck in a fear state has lost her innate sense of trust in the world.

Signs of fear

- May appear very still outwardly but be emotionally agitated

- A tendency to catastrophise and fear the worst

- Voice may have a monotonous, groaning quality to it

Anger

The emotion of anger resonates with the Wood Element. Anger is said to make the *qi* of the Wood Element rise. It has a strong upward moving effect and is an intensely *yang* emotion. However, a one-off experience of intense anger is unlikely to have any long-term effect on the flow of *qi* in a child.

Anger becomes detrimental when it is unexpressed, perhaps even unrecognised, within the child. Rather than causing a temporary upward movement of *qi*, it then means the *qi* of the Wood Element becomes constrained or stagnant. This may manifest as either chronic irritability or frustration.

Often, however, it manifests as depression, which is sometimes described as 'frozen rage'. The *yang*, dynamic *qi* of the Wood Element has become stuck and imploded, meaning the child will often feel that life is hopeless, there is no point in anything and she cannot be bothered.

Signs of internalised anger

- Tiredness that is not relieved by sleep

- A strong 'can't be bothered' or 'what's the point?' attitude

- Feels better for exercise and movement

- Body looks and feels tense and rigid

- Voice is clipped or shouting

Shock

Strictly speaking, shock is not a single emotion, but it disrupts the entire emotional system of a child. Consequently, it is extremely detrimental to a child's fragile *shen*. Shock is synonymous with trauma. It resonates with both the Fire and the Water Element, and tends to disrupt the flow of *qi* between these two Elements. The balance between Fire (*yang*) and Water (*yin*) is a pivot around which the stability of a child's mental/emotional health rests. So when this balance is disturbed, it is as if the core of mental/emotional stability is compromised. The influential physician Zhang Jiebin wrote that after a shock 'the spirits are frightened, and they disperse'.[1] According to Chinese medicine, the child's *qi* 'scatters', like birds when a bird of prey swoops in. A child is particularly susceptible to shock, because her *qi* is volatile and not yet robust. We will discuss the effects of shock in more detail in Chapter 11, 'Times of Change'.

> Nine-year-old Elise came to my acupuncture clinic for treatment. Since being bitten by a dog a couple of months ago, she had begun to burst into tears for no apparent reason several times a day. This was very uncharacteristic of her. It was the way she manifested the shock of her experience with the dog.

Signs of shock

Shock can manifest in a multitude of different ways. There is often an initial strong, physical reaction to shock, such as incontinence of bowels or bladder, shaking or loss of speech. In the longer term, signs of past shock may include:

- jumpiness

- pale face

- emotional volatility

- poor sleep

- the child does not 'feel herself' any more.

A NOTE ABOUT DESIRE

Desire is not one of the seven emotions talked about in the Chinese medical classics. However, it is considered detrimental by all three key Chinese philosophies: Daoism, Confucianism and Buddhism. It is said to stir up *heat* in the body which then rises and agitates the *shen*. So in that way it can trigger anxious feelings.

Many children today live in a constant state of desire. They are bombarded by advertisements which lead them to believe that only when they have the latest pair of trainers, the newest smart phone or the perfect body, will they be happy. We talk more about desire in Chapter 12, 'The *Yin* and *Yang* of Daily Life'.

Two and two don't always make four

It is easy to slip into assuming that a particular event will cause a particular emotion in a child. However, emotional responses are entirely individual and determined by many different factors, an important one being the Element type of the child.

One child who has been on the receiving end of some bullying behaviour at school may have a *yin* response, feeling upset and tearful. Another might have a more *yang* response, and feel real fury towards the child who has been bullying. Yet another child might have a fear response to the same situation. We should try to be curious about a child's emotional responses rather than making assumptions.

A family with five children are sitting down eating their supper one night, when Mum and Dad make a big announcement. Mum has a new job and they are leaving the city where they have always lived and moving to a different one hundreds of miles away. Each of the five children has a different response.

The Fire child begins to cry and says, 'If you really loved me, you wouldn't make me move. I can't bear to leave all my friends behind.'

The Earth child doesn't eat her supper and by bedtime that evening is fraught with worry. 'Who will pick me up from school if you have a new job, Mum? And I might not even like my new school, and the teachers might not be kind.' Her list of worries goes on and on until she wears herself out and eventually falls asleep.

The Metal child goes quiet. She becomes a bit withdrawn over the next few weeks, but her parents struggle to draw her out over what she is feeling.

The Water child becomes quite agitated and immediately imagines the worst-case scenario. She says, 'We'll never find a house as nice as this one. I bet Grandma will get ill again and we won't be here to help her. And what happens if your new job doesn't work out and then we are stuck there forever for no good reason?'

The Wood child gets up from the table and pushes her chair over. She goes red in the face and shouts, 'How could you do this? I don't want to move. I hate you both.'

Although (as the example above shows) each Element type will have a tendency towards a particular emotion, there are no black and white rules. Just because you know a particular child is a Wood type, it would be a mistake to assume her emotional response will always be anger. The key is always to be curious, observe and respond according to what you find, rather than what you think you are going to find.

Repressing or disconnecting from emotions

As we have seen, each emotion resonates with a particular Element (or, as in the case of sadness and shock, more than one Element). All five Elements are connected, which means that the emotions are connected too. This means that if there is difficulty with one emotion, there is likely to be difficulty with another. The most common way this manifests is that when a child disconnects from or represses an emotion, it prevents them from being able to feel other emotions. For example, disconnecting from feeling anger will make it difficult to feel joyful.

However, almost the opposite is also true. Repressing an emotion because it is too uncomfortable to fully experience can mean that the child expresses another emotion instead. For example, trying to escape feelings of sadness might mean that anxiety comes in its place. Not acknowledging fear might mean that anger is expressed in its place. So:

- disconnecting from one emotion can result in a child not being able to feel others

- disconnecting from one emotion can result in a child feeling another in its place.

The Disney-Pixar movie *Inside Out* illustrates beautifully how emotions are all interlinked. Riley, the protagonist, moves to a new city and has an awful time of it. She has lost all her joy and can't get back to it. She will not admit to herself or anybody else that she feels sad. With the help of her imaginary childhood friend, Bing Bong, Riley gets in touch with her sadness and expresses the fact that she misses her old city and life to her parents. Once she has acknowledged and verbalised this feeling, her joy is able to find a way back in and she continues her new life in a much better frame of mind, experiencing all her emotions more fluidly.

Picking up on others' emotions

It is not only her own emotional responses that a child has to contend with. She will also be affected by others' emotions. As we mentioned in Chapter 2, a child's *qi* is not yet consolidated so she is especially sensitive to her emotional environment. She is a bit like a smoke alarm that goes off when you put the toaster on in the morning. Her *qi* will react to everything. Obviously the degree to which this happens depends on the individual's constitution, but as a general rule children are particularly inclined to this kind of sensitivity.

For example, parents have often told me that ever since their child joined a new class at school, she has seemed to come home angry and take it out on her little brother. If I enquire about the nature of the new teacher, it turns out she is what the child calls a 'shouty' teacher. The child has absorbed the teacher's angry *qi* during the day and then manifests it at home after school.

Another parent told me how his son would invariably come home from staying with his grandparents hyped up and unable to sleep. When I enquired about the grandparents, it turned out that they were both super-high achievers who had a tendency to be rather adrenalised and competitive.

The connection between the seven emotions and anxiety and depression

In Chapter 6, we discussed the fact that anxiety and depression are catch-all terms for a wide variety of different states. If we can help a child to connect with the original emotion, and support him to find ways of managing that emotion, then the anxiety and the low feelings are likely to recede. Having read this chapter, I hope that you will now be able to develop a better understanding of a particular child's emotional state. One child's so-called depression might be more accurately described as imploded anger. Another child's anxiety might be a substitute for a deep feeling of sadness.

Lilly started to feel anxious when she was nine. Her anxiety spiked on a Sunday night but had become almost constant. Lilly struggled to articulate what she was anxious about. She described feeling on edge and felt she could never relax. At first, her parents were baffled as to what had caused the anxiety, as there had been no obvious trigger and as a young child Lilly hadn't shown any propensity at all to being anxious. They mentioned that, on the contrary, even when Lilly's closest, lifelong friend had seemingly overnight rejected her in favour of another girl, Lilly had seemed to take it in her stride.

Lilly's demeanour appeared to me to be more one of anger than anxiety. I also noticed that her voice sounded rather clipped and as if she was always shouting. Over a period of time, Lilly began to talk about her friend, and her feelings of fury that she blanked her whenever their paths crossed at school, as if they had never known each other. The more she expressed her anger, the less anxious she became. In time, and with the help of acupuncture, she got back her spark and began enjoying life a lot more, free of both anger and sadness.

WHAT CAN WE DO TO HELP?
Step 1: being an emotion detective

- With close observation, begin to try to get a sense of the emotion underlying a child's anxiety or depression.

  - Does her face reveal a particular emotion when she is in repose?

- Does her body reveal any clues? It might be tight, or her shoulders might be hunched, for example.

- Does the tone of her voice convey a particular emotion?

- What emotions are evoked in you when you are around the child?

- Were there any big events in the child's life in the time before she became anxious or depressed? What was her response to those? Did a powerful emotion get buried at that time?

- Is there an emotion that is taboo in the family? What emotion does the child feel it is not acceptable to admit to?

Step 2: coaxing the emotion into the open

- Saying something like 'I wonder if you are feeling sad about that' or 'I guess that might have made you angry' can help a child to identify what she is feeling. It's a fine line between guiding a child and leading the witness though.

- Showing a child a range of emojis and asking her to point to the one that matches how she is feeling can be a useful tool.

- With an older child, non-threatening and compassionate enquiry can help her to name what she is feeling. There are certain key elements for this to be successful:

  - The child needs to feel the adult is not going to respond emotionally to what she reveals.

  - The child needs to feel that what she says will not be belittled or denied (e.g. if she says she feels worried she is going to flunk her exams, responding with 'Oh, you don't need to worry, you will pass with flying colours' denies her feelings and will hinder her chances of being able to process them).

  - The child needs to feel emotionally 'held' and safe in order to reveal how she is feeling.

  - Any sense of being rushed or pressured to reveal something will backfire.

Step 3: sitting with the emotion

- Bringing an emotion up to the surface eventually gives it less power. However, in the short term, it can be uncomfortable or even excruciating, which is probably why the child pushed the emotion away in the first place.

- Having an adult who can be truly present, listen without judgement if the child wants to verbalise her feelings or otherwise just be alongside the child while she experiences them can help the child allow her feelings to come up to the surface.

- When a child is struggling to manage an intense feeling, there are various practical steps that can support her:

  - simple breathing exercises (see Chapter 14)

  - holding and playing with a squishy

  - movement (walking, yoga, stretching...)

  - cuddling an animal

  - having a comfort toy to hand

  - being with a trusted adult.

Step 4: dissipating the emotion

- One reason a child may push down an emotion is because it remains intense over a long period of time. It is too strong for her to bear. So helping an emotion to dissipate and become unstuck is the next step. The aim here is definitely not to push the emotion back down, or make it go away, but to lessen the intensity and help it to flow. Please see Appendix 4 for suggestions for how to do this.

Seeing the wood for the trees

- ▶ In Chinese medicine, emotions are simply understood to be movements of *qi*.

- ▶ Different emotions induce the *qi* to move in a particular way.

- ▸ If an emotion is intense, prolonged or repressed, it means the *qi* of the child cannot regain its equilibrium, and it will become disordered.

- ▸ Once *qi* becomes disordered, it makes it harder for emotions to flow freely within a child.

- ▸ When emotions are prevented from flowing freely, anxiety and depression are more likely to take hold.

- ▸ Chinese medicine talks of seven 'key' emotions, any of which may be the underlying cause of a child being anxious or depressed.

- ▸ Depending on a child's Five Element constitution, he will respond to life events with his own, particular emotional nuance.

- ▸ The key is to *observe* a child and to *be curious*.

Endnote

1   C. Larre and E. Rochat de la Vallée (1995) *Rooted in Spirit* (New York: Station Hill Press), p. 127.

• Chapter 9 •

Connection

The big picture

We all know that feeling connected to others tends to make us happier. It is incontrovertible that having good relationships is one of the strongest contributory factors to a long and happy life. Human interaction is actually life-saving for babies. For toddlers and children, it is a key ingredient for healthy growth and development. For teens, good relationships are key to maintaining psychological health. In short, connection, intimacy and good relationships are a key protective factor against anxiety and depression.

Yet as well as being one of the most crucial aspects of our lives, relationships remain one of the most challenging. A sleep-deprived mother whose baby cries every minute he is awake may have to dig deep to remain connected to her feelings of love for her child. How can siblings' love for each other not be diminished by their feelings of competitiveness for the attention of their hardworking parent? It can be really difficult for a ten-year-old girl who changes to a new school to form relationships with girls who have known each other for years already. Some of the most challenging relationships are between teens and their parents. The teen just wants freedom and the parent feels fearful of letting go. At different times, and for a variety of reasons, connection can be difficult.

Connection is not a one-off event, but an ongoing process. Children need connection of different forms at different times of their lives. A child not only needs to have connection with others throughout childhood; he also needs to be supported in how to create and maintain relationships of different kinds as he goes through life.

Chinese medicine's unique perspective and language can help us to understand why relationships are so important, how to make them better and, crucially, how they help to protect against anxiety and depression.

● THE PAST CANNOT BE CHANGED

The focus of the first part of this chapter is on the early weeks and months of life. If you are reading this as the parent of an older child or teenager who is struggling, you may feel anxious yourself or hopeless that it is too late to help your child. You may berate yourself for not having been a perfect parent in the earlier years of your child's life. If that is the case, I would like to reassure you.

First, while it is true that the early years are influential, it is never too late to help a child. A child or teen is a work in progress. Her *qi* is not yet 'set' and therefore it is much easier to bring about a lasting change in her mental/emotional state than it is with an adult. Second, when is life ever perfect? And is there really such a thing as perfect anyway? Most of us reach adulthood in reasonable psychological shape despite our imperfect childhoods. One thing you can be absolutely sure of is that berating yourself for something that cannot be changed does not help your child. Of course, reflecting on the past is important, as it can help us to make the present and the future better. You may even feel you can have a conversation with an older child about times when you struggled to be the parent you wanted to be. However, the present is the place that deserves most of our focus when it comes to building connection with a child.

The key points

- Human connection is a protective factor against childhood anxiety and depression.

- Human connection affects the balance of *yin/yang* within a child, as well as the way her *qi* and the Five Elements develop.

- Human connection takes place on many different levels and via many different pathways.

How to connect
Connecting through the eyes

The well-known proverb states that 'The eyes are the window to the soul.' Chinese medicine has always stressed the importance of looking at the eyes to diagnose the state of the person's *shen*. A healthy *shen* will manifest with bright and sparkling eyes. At the same time, connection with others (which feeds the *shen*) is achieved in part through eye contact. When a baby first smiles and looks into the eyes of her main caregiver, which is usually sometime around the age of three months, her *shen* comes alive. In order to promote the development of the *shen*, a baby needs reciprocity. When she looks into her mother's eyes, she needs to see that there is a response. These little moments of eye contact are the seeds of how the baby learns about connection and relationships. It is the equivalent of learning the alphabet before she learns how to read and write. They are a fundamental building block that will influence the ability and ease with which she manages relationships as she grows.

On the one hand, for a parent to look into his baby's eyes and have these moments of intense connection seems so fundamental to being a parent that it hardly needs mention. On the other, the stress of being a new parent and the worry of 'getting it right' can mean that it is easy for parents to think that other things are more important. One mother, who was reflecting on the difficult months after her first child was born, said she now felt sad because she had been so preoccupied with making sure her baby was putting on weight, getting into a routine and meeting his developmental milestones that she overlooked simply enjoying being in the presence of her baby.

Connecting through *qi*

Connection also happens when we are not actively interacting with a baby. As adults, we all recognise the difference between sitting in silence with someone to whom we feel no connection compared with someone to whom we feel close. The former can mean we feel uneasy, alone and perhaps anxious. The latter can bring about a feeling of togetherness and calm.

A baby can sense whether a parent is purely physically present rather than being physically *and* emotionally present. When a parent or caregiver is truly present, they are able to tune in to their baby and respond to her needs from moment to moment. The *qi* of the baby and the caregiver merge with each other and are in a constant interchange. The baby will then feel connected and safe. This creates an environment in which her *shen* can more easily thrive. The more a parent is able to be present in mind, body and spirit (rather than just body), the more connected a baby will feel to her.

Connecting through touch

One very important means of forming connection is touch. Of course, touch is often an instinctual part of the relationship between a parent and young child. However, it is something that many children, especially as they grow older, do not get enough of. Busy family lives mean there is less time for a close and loving physical relationship with children.

So, why is touch such an important protective factor against anxiety and depression?

A permeable membrane

In Chinese medicine, the skin and touch are related to the Metal Element. The Metal Element gives a child his instinct for protection. It provides a kind of barrier or membrane between the child's body and his external environment. Ideally, he will feel connected to and affected by what goes on around him, but he will be neither over-protected nor overly exposed.

For example, if the membrane is insufficient he may feel especially vulnerable to criticism. The harsh words of a ragged parent at bedtime might feel as if they penetrate right to the core of his being. His degree of upset might, to the parent, feel exaggerated in response to the trigger. On the other hand, if the membrane is too thick, he may be somewhat closed off, be hard to contact and may appear unmoved by events in his life that we might expect to induce emotion. For the child, to be in this state may feel isolating.

The right kind of touch can help to regulate the child's membrane. It can promote balance so that a child is adequately, but not overly, protected from outside influences.

Eight-year-old Amy was adopted at age two, and had spent the first two years of her life in an orphanage where she barely received any physical touch. She struggled with sensory processing issues, which are often a result of the membrane not having developed properly. She was hypersensitive to noise and spent most of the day with her hands over her ears, trying to block out even run-of-the-mill noises. However, she barely seemed to register the sensation of touch. She had an upsetting habit of digging her nails deep into her skin, as she said it was the only way she could actually feel something.

Amy was brought to my acupuncture clinic. I treated her with non-needling methods which involve light stroking over particular parts of the body. I also gave her mother a series of Chinese medicine massages to do at home every day, focusing on the particular imbalance in Amy's *qi*. Over time, Amy began to be able to tolerate noise more easily and her need to dig her nails into her skin lessened. Her skin membrane became more regulated.

Ready for battle

When a child feels under stress, the body will respond by readying itself for battle. From a Chinese medicine perspective, one way of doing this is by sending its resources to the surface of the body. This is akin to sending troops to the front in preparation to defend against potential attackers. This is a useful response when there really is a threat. However, to live in a constant state of red-alert means the child can never fully switch off and relax. It is also simply tiring to be in this state for any length of time. The right kind of touch can help to 'de-stress' a child by signalling that a threat is no longer present. This will help them to achieve a more relaxed state.

Touch is especially important for young babies because it is the primary way in which they experience the world. However, touch is beneficial for children and teens too. It becomes harder for parents to find acceptable ways of touching their teenage children. However, when the moment presents itself, it should be taken. With a teen, sometimes a hug at bedtime or a foot massage when he is stressed about exams is an easier way of keeping connection than with words.

WHAT CAN WE DO TO HELP?

Here are some suggestions for ways of making sure babies and children of different ages have touch in their lives:

For parents

- Skin to skin contact for babies.

- Safe co-sleeping in the early years.

- Carrying babies in slings rather than pushing them in buggies.

- Baby massage.

- Including small moments of loving touch as part of day-to-day life, e.g. pats on the shoulder, hugs and cuddles.

- Touch does not need to be limited to humans – cuddling and stroking animals is a great way for kids to increase their daily touch quota.

For practitioners

- Incorporating touch-based modalities into our treatments of young people is a wonderful tool to help lower anxiety levels and lift mood. Even children who find unplanned touch difficult can enjoy and respond well to the intentional touch of paediatric *tui na* or *shonishin*. Beyond their medical effects, these methods have the additional benefits of regulating the membrane at the surface of the body.

Connecting through words

As a baby grows into a toddler and then a child, connection and intimacy are created through words too. In Chinese medicine, speech is understood to be governed by the *shen* and the Heart. The *shen* and the Heart influence a child's ability to communicate verbally. In turn, verbal communication nourishes the *shen* and the Heart. Anxiety often involves an imbalance of the *shen* and the Heart organ. Talking, therefore, really is powerful. It is not just the content of what is said that provides benefits but the very act of talking itself. Talking is a means by which a child's *shen* finds expression in the world.

Taking time to listen as a child begins to express himself through words, repeating back to him what he has said or answering his many 'why' questions helps a child's *shen* to thrive, nourishes his Heart and therefore helps him to feel connected. It is upsetting to see a parent and child in cafes and restaurants not talking to each other, usually because one or both of them are looking at a screen of some sort. In these instances, we are only seeing a snapshot of a relationship, and of course it is not reasonable to expect a parent and their child to be constantly talking. However, conversation is a key tool in remaining connected as a child grows. It is also an art that needs to be developed from a young age, rather than something a child will automatically be able to do with no practice. Developing this art therefore equips a child with a key skill to help him build connections with others, thereby serving as a protective factor against anxiety and depression.

Every child has her own language of connection

Every child will have her own way of experiencing connection. As a parent or practitioner, we should not assume that the way *we* make our connections with people is the only way. The Five Element system is a really helpful lens through which to understand how we might best connect with an individual child. You might want to check back to Chapter 5, to remind yourself of the differing needs of each Element type.

Who a child connects with
Connections outside the family

The family is the early learning ground for a baby and small child to discover how to connect with others and communicate. In the Chinese medicine texts, there are lots of warnings about the importance of keeping strangers out of the home of a young baby and avoiding exposing her to too many outside influences. While we should not take this too literally, the idea being conveyed is that, in the realm of relationships, children should not be expected to run before they can walk. Once a child feels secure and connected to her primary caregivers and other close family members, her next challenge is to practise connecting with a wider circle of people.

There is an African proverb which goes 'it takes a village to raise a child.' It reveals the importance of children being part of a community, rather than just a family. I like to equate it with a plant needing a bigger pot as it grows. If it were to stay in a small pot, there would not be enough soil, or enough nutrients in the soil, to carry on supporting the plant's best growth. The more varied and meaningful connections a child has, the more nourishment there is available for his *shen*. A wider circle of connections also allows a child more space for his *shen* to bloom and blossom. Even the happiest family can feel a little claustrophobic and constraining at times.

The way in which each child approaches connecting with others will be heavily influenced by her constitutional nature. For example, a gregarious Fire child may relish the opportunity to go to a children's party where there are lots of potential new friends. An introverted Metal child, on the other hand, may find that experience overwhelming. So, one of the most important ways to support a child in creating connections outside the family is to try to understand and acknowledge the unique challenges that may be involved for each particular child.

Connections in the teenage years

This brings us to the teenage years. We will discuss adolescence more in Chapter 11. There are two important points to make here. The first is that **teenagers need friends**. More specifically, they need connections outside the family and to find a tribe (other than their family) to which they feel connected. The second is that, although this may not appear to be the case, **teenagers need to feel connected to family**. It might be helpful to explain this in terms of *yin/yang*.

Connection and closeness with family members meets a teenager's *yin* needs – for safety, security, nurture and constancy. Connection and closeness with friends and a new tribe outside of the family meets a teenager's *yang* needs – for expansion, exploration and independence. One without the other creates an imbalance. If a teen is either struggling to make friends for some reason, or has a parent who does not find it easy to loosen the reins, he will have no way of expressing the *yang* part of him. If, on the other hand, a teen is out and about with his friends all the time, and he does not have a secure and connected family base to go back to, he will have no way of nurturing his *yin*. Figure 9.1 illustrates the *yin/yang* needs of adolescent connection.

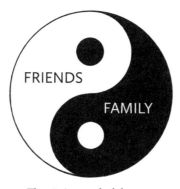

Figure 9.1 The yin/yang of adolescent connection

It can also be really difficult for parents to remain connected to their teens, even when they have been close up to that point. Below are some suggestions for ways to help this process.

● WHAT CAN WE DO TO HELP?

- Much of the time, teens are working hard at becoming independent. If a parent asks for connection at the time of her choosing, it may be experienced by the teen as restraint. Parents of a teen will benefit from being *yin* and showing flexibility, so they are ready to relate at the time of their child's choosing.

- Teens often find it easier to relate when they are doing something or being active, in other words, when they are expressing their *yang*. Finding an activity that the teen enjoys and that the parent can share with them is a great opportunity for connecting.

- Although parents might fear that allowing their teen more freedom and independence will mean less connection, the opposite is often true. The less a teen feels constrained, the more free-flowing his *qi* will be. Free-flowing *qi* promotes connection.

In order to connect with a child, we need to listen to them. Listening is not a passive activity. The traditional Chinese character for listening includes the symbols for not only the ears, but the eyes and the heart, indicating that it is a multi-sensory experience. The fact that it contains the symbol for the heart is of particular interest. It suggests that, when we listen, what we hear resonates with our own inner world. Listening is, therefore, a two-way, connection-building process.

Connection with the self

So far in this chapter, we have been talking about the importance of connecting with others, the fact that this nourishes a child's *shen*. However, there is another connection that is equally important, and that is a child's connection with herself. There are two aspects of this.

Ming – individual destiny

In China there is a concept known as *ming*, which is usually translated as 'individual destiny'. As well as enabling a child to connect with others, the *shen* also guides a child towards her *ming,* i.e. along a path that is uniquely suited to her. It helps her to act in a way which makes sense according to her own distinctive nature and the context of her environment. It provides a guiding light so that the child can manifest her unique potential in the world. This is a *yang* aspect of the *shen.*

Ling – the inner self

However, there is a *yin* aspect of the *shen* too. This is called the *ling* and refers to the more hidden, inner parts of a child's spirit that cannot be perceived through the eyes and are not so obvious to the world. The *ling* is an important concept in any discussion of anxiety and depression. These states are more likely to arise when a child is not familiar or comfortable with the more hidden parts of her being. When a child is beset by anxious thoughts, it can be helpful to ponder what she would be thinking or feeling otherwise. Sometimes, the answer is that she would be experiencing emotions and plagued by thoughts which are more uncomfortable than her anxieties.

In order for a child to begin to know himself and to become acquainted with the more hidden realms of his inner world, he needs to have times of stillness. He needs opportunities for his focus to be turned inwards rather than directed outwards towards his external environment. Knowing oneself is a key protective factor against anxiety and depression. As Socrates wisely said, 'An unexamined life is not worth living'.

Fifteen-year-old Zara had spent much of her free time, since the age of seven, playing several musical instruments to a high level. She practised for hours each day, performed in her school orchestra and had also won a place in a prestigious county youth orchestra. Her parents were very happy about this, particularly her mother, who was a talented musician herself.

Zara was known as 'the musical one' in the family and at school. For birthdays and Christmas, her relatives would always give her mu-sic-related presents. She had been quite happy with this and enjoyed the admiration she got for having reached such high standards in all her instruments.

However, seemingly overnight, at the age of fifteen, Zara had an acute episode of severe low mood and quite extreme anxiety. It took her some months of feeling like this to get to the bottom of the problem: she did not enjoy playing her instruments any more.

It took great courage for Zara to admit this, both to herself and to others. Her identity had been so closely tied with being 'the musical one'. However, once she had acknowledged it, over time she began to feel happy again and less anxious. She then began filling her time with a range of other activities, seeing her friends and sometimes doing simple activities, such as walking the dog.

She reflected that she had never truly enjoyed spending hours a day playing but that because she had been told she was good at it, it was something she just ended up doing. As Zara connected with her true self, her *shen* began to flourish and her symptoms went away.

WHAT CAN WE DO TO HELP?

For parents

Ask yourself the following questions, in relation to the child you have in mind:

- How often are you truly present with your child? This means time when your focus is entirely on her. It is much more about quality than it is quantity. Aim to include some time every day (whatever feels realistic given your circumstances) when your focus is 100 per cent aimed at connecting with your child.

- Are you tending to the connections in your own life? You cannot expect yourself to be really available to connect with a child if your own connection bucket is running dry. Your child will benefit from you tending to your own needs.

- Do you and your child have time in which you can connect? Busyness is the enemy of intimacy. Too hectic a schedule (both your own and your child's) can, on its own, be a barrier to creating connection.

- Are the expectations you have of your parenting too high? The saying goes that perfection is the enemy of the good, but it is also the enemy of connection. Aim to be authentic, rather than perfect.

For practitioners

- Beyond the power of the acupuncture or whichever modality a practitioner uses, the connection we make with a child in the treatment room is of therapeutic value itself. Not being a family member can be an advantage, as there are fewer emotional complexities which can block the connection.

Seeing the wood for the trees

▶ Connection is made through eye contact.

▶ Parents and children are connected through their *qi*.

▶ Touch is a powerful way of promoting connection.

▶ Conversation is an important way of promoting and maintaining connection as a child grows.

▶ Children need connection with an ever-widening circle as they grow older.

▶ During adolescence, teens have a strong need for connection with friends, but connection with family is also crucial.

▶ Children need to be encouraged to remain connected with themselves, as well as with others.

▶ Adults need to respond to the unique nature of each child and find a way of connecting that makes sense to that child.

Chapter 10

Family

The big picture

It was Tolstoy who wrote that 'Happy families are all alike; every unhappy family is unhappy in its own way.' Much as I hate to disagree with one of my literary heroes, it would be more accurate to say that no two families are alike, whether happy or not, even if they appear to be so on the surface. The dynamics within a family are as unique as the individuals who make up that family. Furthermore, most people would probably say that their family life played more of a role in shaping who they became than any other single factor. What goes on in a family creates emotions in a child. If these emotions become intense or prolonged, they disturb the movements of *qi* and can potentially contribute to a child becoming anxious and/or depressed.

No place for blame

Does this mean that a family causes a child to become anxious or depressed? Does it mean that family are to blame for a child's emotional struggles? The answer to that is a categorical 'no'. Or rather, those are just not the right questions to ask. They assume a straightforward causal relationship. The reality is more subtle and more complex. In the vast majority of cases, parents and other family members are doing the best job they possibly can, usually in imperfect circumstances, to love and raise their children. Parents and other adults are all a product of their own imperfect histories. They are linked to and influenced by previous generations, who may have endured personal or external struggles that hugely shaped their ability to parent. It is not as straightforward as the poet Philip Larkin made out: 'They f*** you up, your mum and dad'. It is a child's response to his parents and to what goes on in his family that shapes him. This response is largely shaped by a child's Element type.

Of course, there are some tragic cases when a parent acts in a way that irrevocably harms their child (as in the case of physical, emotional or sexual abuse). However, what normally shapes a child is his unique response to who his family members are and how he interacts with them. In China, there is an understanding that it is the relationship between things that is more important than the individual things themselves. An individual's psychological problems, for example, are usually seen as being problems *in relation to* other individuals (especially other family members), rather than problems arising *because of* other individuals.

The key point here is to avoid playing the 'blame game'. Family members (as we will discuss in more detail below) are all intimately connected to one another. Sometimes, a dynamic between two or more of them develops that influences the child emotionally. Nobody has caused this, and nobody wanted it to happen. It just is. The most fruitful response is to take a step back, watch, notice and reflect on this dynamic. Bringing it more into consciousness immediately begins to lessen its power. We will discuss later in this chapter some tools to help you do this.

The Chinese medicine view
Treat the mother to heal the child

'Treat the mother to treat the child' (*zhi mu yi zhi zi*) is a common and important saying in Chinese medicine. The word 'mother' here applies not just to the biological mother, but to a child's main caregiver in the early months of their lives, whichever gender. I am going to use the word 'mother' for simplicity's sake, and because in the majority of families it is still the mother who is most likely to take on the role of main caregiver.

In Chinese medicine, the mother and baby are understood to function as a unit for the first years of a child's life, and their *qi* is regarded as being intertwined. As is the case with *yin* and *yang*, mother and child are interdependent. A child actually receives *qi* from his mother. This will happen regardless of whether the child is breastfed or not. A baby needs more than just milk to survive. His essential needs extend beyond mere nutrients, and include touch, interaction and simply the presence of loving caregivers. All of these things help to nurture and feed his *qi*, so that he develops strongly.

So, why is this important? Most parents recognise that their young child's mood is often a reflection of their own mood on a particular day. When you are stressed and irritable, your child is more likely to be fractious and grumpy. When you are exhausted, your child may be more clingy and demanding. On days when you are at your most relaxed or energetic, your child may follow suit. However, this mirroring of emotions and behaviour between parent and child does not only take place from moment to moment but also on a more long-term basis. The child of a chronically anxious mother will imbibe the anxiety and it becomes his own. A vicious circle is created: having an anxious child often increases the mother's anxiety.

There is another factor to this relationship which, in reality, is not quite as simple as the above description. This is, of course, the unique emotional nature of the child. For example, the Wood child's emotional response to having an anxious mother might be anger. The Metal child's response to having an anxious mother might be to feel that he is lacking ('If I were a better child, Mum would be happier'). Or the child of a very anxious parent may become particularly reckless in the teenage years.

One of the most effective actions an adult caregiver can take to help a child who is feeling anxious or depressed is to prioritise and work on managing his or her own emotions. The advantage of the fact that a mother's and a child's *qi* are so connected is that it is possible for the mother to almost do the emotional work on behalf of her child, especially in the early years.

The aim is not perfection. Having a range of emotions is only human, and a child will benefit from witnessing a wide range of emotions in the adults who care for them. The most crucial thing is for the parent to avoid getting 'stuck' in one emotion.

It is impossible to overemphasise the worry and anxiety that having a child who is struggling with her mental/emotional health will cause in a parent. Just as a child is heavily impacted by the emotions of her parent, the same is true the other way around. However, it is always the parents who should set the emotional tone for the family. It is therefore even more important for the parent of an anxious or depressed child to be tending to their own emotional state.

WHAT CAN WE DO TO HELP?

We've talked a lot about how every child is unique, but, as adults, we are unique too. So everyone needs to find a method or methods of managing their emotions that best suits them. Some suggestions are:

- working on your relationships with partners, family and friends

- acupuncture

- talking therapy

- exercise

- creating more time in your schedule

- lessening your commitments

- looking after your physical health through diet and sleep.

Everyone is interlinked

It is not only the mother and child who are interlinked. All the members of a family are interdependent. In an ideal world, they will be intimately connected, yet there will be space for each person to express his individuality. A family member should feel part of a unit but also accepted for who he is. Ideally, there will be an unspoken knowing that when one member is struggling, the others will step up and take the strain. There will be enough dynamism to allow for the balance between the members to shift as they grow and change.

This idea of how a family system works mirrors the way that the Five Elements are connected and work together. As shown in Figure 1.4, each Element is connected to each of the other four. In Chinese medicine, we understand that what happens to and within one Element will have a knock-on impact on each of the other four. This also happens within a family. To quote a renowned living practitioner of Chinese medicine, Liu Yousheng, 'The Five Elements all affect each other, and if the Five Elements do not function smoothly within the family, this naturally affects the way the Five Elements function within the human body.'[1]

So, having established that everyone in a family is inextricably linked, what does this actually mean for a child's mental/emotional health? It means that a child's anxiety and/or depression may be partly a result of some dysfunction within the family system. So, rather than the focus being purely on the child who is having emotional difficulties, it is often worth putting the child's struggles within the context of the family and bringing about a shift in the dynamics of the family. In my paediatric acupuncture clinic, I take the view that even though the child may be the one ostensibly coming for treatment, in a sense the whole family are in the treatment room.

Sometimes, a child becomes the emotional scapegoat of the family. Unwittingly, it is as if the other family members hand over all their difficult emotions to the child. The child, because of her sensitivity and her Element type, takes on the emotions and they lead her to feel anxious and/or depressed. She acts like a sponge and soaks up the problems within the family. It is almost as if her doing this enables the rest of the family unit to keep functioning. It is easy for a family to fall into thinking, 'We're all fine – Jane is the one with the problem.' Of course, most of this goes on at an unconscious level.

There is a story that illustrates this concept of the emotional scapegoat in a lovely book by the psychoanalyst Stephen Grosz, called *The Examined Life*. A ten-year-old girl who was brought to him for therapy because she wet herself both day and night was chaotic, messy and dishevelled. The rest of her family were all exceptionally well dressed, high-achieving and 'together'. Grosz writes that, over the year he was seeing the girl, she gradually began to put her hair up and generally take more care over her appearance, as well as stopping having accidents. He also noted that, at the same time, the other members of her family who brought her to the clinic became more scruffy and chaotic. His receptionist pointed out to him that 'It happens a lot here – as the children get well, their families change too.'[2]

HOW THE *QI* OF FAMILY MEMBERS IS INTERLINKED

Isaac, a ten-year-old boy, was suffering from extreme anxiety. His mother told me that Isaac's father worked relentlessly hard because he was fearful that he would otherwise be made redundant. Even his hard work did not pay off as he did indeed lose his job. As is often the case, however, sometimes the thing we most fear turns out to be not so bad. Within a couple of months, Isaac's father had found a new job working for a company who did not expect him to be superhuman and where he felt safe and secure. The real silver lining to the story is that, at the same time, Isaac's anxiety disappeared almost overnight.

● WHAT CAN WE DO TO HELP?

This is a simple exercise that might help bring to the surface some underlying family dynamics that are contributing to a child's poor mental/emotional health.

On a big sheet of paper, draw a circle for each family member and write their name inside the circle. Beside each circle, make a note of any obvious strains that person is carrying. For example, you might write 'chronic back pain/grieving for mother who died last year/ongoing conflict with sibling' next to the mother's circle, or 'struggling with friendships/self-conscious about acne/big exams looming' next to the teenage brother's circle.

You might be surprised to see that the child manifesting the anxiety and/or depression is not the one who has the long list of obvious strains beside his circle.

Reflect on what your picture reveals and reassess where you need to focus your help and support. It might be that supporting one member of the family reduces the anxiety and/or depression of another member.

The fit between family members

If you were to ask siblings to describe their family life as a child, you would probably hear surprisingly different stories. Some of this can be accounted for by the fact that each sibling truly did have a different experience, perhaps because of a large age gap, or one being sent off to boarding school and another staying at home. However, the most likely reason for the different perceptions is that each child absorbed a different experience due to their own emotional natures. The child psychologist Donald Winnicott explained that each sibling in a family will experience their mother differently (and the mother will reveal different parts of herself to each of her children).

How, you may ask, might this contribute to a child feeling anxious and/or depressed?

A child may not get her core emotional needs met because of a mismatch between the way her parents express their love for their child and the way she receives it, which is largely dependent on her Element type. I will illustrate this by giving some examples:

Gerry is a thirteen-year-old Wood child who feels loved when he is trusted and given a lot of independence. Gerry's mother is an Earth type who has a propensity to worry. Her worry leads her to keep Gerry close. Gerry feels constrained and angry as a result of this. He does not express his anger and frustration, which then implode and lead him to feel depressed.

Laura is a nine-year-old Water child. She is very sensitive and loves to spend time at home drawing and painting. Laura's parents are both Wood types whose idea of a good weekend is to go out hiking, climbing and kayaking. They really want Laura to join them in their activities and think she will benefit a lot from doing them. Laura easily feels scared and becomes over-adrenalised when she joins these outdoor pursuits. She comes home feeling agitated and spends much of the week anxious about what the next weekend holds.

Sammy is a six-year-old Metal child. He is very self-contained and feels easily overwhelmed by lots of hugs and kisses. Sammy's dad is a Fire type who expresses his love for his son through lots of physical affection. He feels a little hurt and rejected when Sammy recoils from his attempts to hug him at bedtime. Over time, this makes Sammy and his dad more distant, and Sammy imbibes the message that there is something 'wrong' with him for not wanting his dad to cuddle him. He feels sad and disconnected from his dad which, as he grows older, makes him prone to depressive episodes.

WHAT CAN WE DO TO HELP?

As a parent, it is helpful to take some time to reflect on how you express your love to your child. Is your way of showing love one that your child can receive? Reflect on an interaction that has not gone well. See if you can put yourself into your child's shoes, based on what you think her Element type is. Did something she did or said trigger an emotional response in you because of your Element type? Picking apart an interaction in this way can help to bring clarity to a difficult emotional dynamic.

THE IMPORTANCE OF UNDERSTANDING A CHILD'S ELEMENT TYPE

Twelve-year-old Jakob and his dad were having a difficult time. Jakob complained that he did not feel that his dad cared about him. Jakob's dad simply could not understand this. He spent most of every weekend helping Jakob with his homework. He frequently suggested they watch wildlife documentaries together, which Jakob's dad had adored when he was Jakob's age. Jakob, a Fire child, responded by saying, 'But I just want to have fun with you, dad! When I go to my friend Fin's house, he and his dad have such a laugh playing rough and tumble together, going out and playing crazy golf or just watching comedy programmes.' When Jakob's dad read about the different Element types, and understood that Jakob was Fire and he was Metal, he had a light-bulb moment. He finally understood why his son, who he poured so much time into and absolutely adored, did not feel loved by him. He told Jakob that every weekend, Jakob could choose something that he wanted to do together, rather than imposing what he thought Jakob would enjoy. From that moment on, Jakob began to feel much closer to his dad and his happiness improved as a result.

Super-scrutiny

A generation ago, families often had many more children than they do now and the world was, perhaps, a less competitive place. There was less perception of 'stranger danger' and less fear of traffic. For these reasons (among others), a more hands-off parenting style was the norm. It was often the case, for example, that children would be sent out of the house after breakfast with a sandwich, and told not to come home before supper time. 'Latchkey kids' were left to their own devices after school while their parents were still out at work. While it is easy to idealise the past, and this hands-off approach probably meant more child neglect, perhaps the pendulum has swung too far the other way.

Many children now have their lives micro-managed for them. Decisions about every aspect are pored over by their parents. What they eat, how they spend their time, which activities they do, what friends they see…the list goes on. This type of parenting has been labelled 'helicopter style', because of the parents' tendency to hover over their children. It can almost be as if the parent is living vicariously through their child.

Sometimes, love and interference become confused. Of course, the degree of involvement a parent has in their child's life must depend on the age, maturity and nature of the child. However, there are very few children, especially as they grow older, who thrive when their life is put under the microscope.

As mentioned previously, the Chinese are more focused on the relationship between things than they are on the individual entities. This applies to the family too. A renowned 19th-century healer called Wang Fengyi talked at length about the fact that the focus of parents should not be on the child, but on harmony within the family. Too much focus on the child, he said, prevents the child from being happy and becoming independent.

Excessive scrutiny affects children in a variety of ways, largely according to their Five Element nature. It rarely, if ever, encourages emotional prosperity. From a *yin/yang* perspective, love, nurture and care can be understood as the *yin* aspect of a child's needs. The *yang* aspect entails space, time and the freedom to experience life, make some mistakes along the way and grow as a result. It is through these *yang* aspects that a child learns to trust that he is fundamentally OK and he develops resilience. He needs to be allowed to 'test his muscles'. A child who is constantly scrutinized is like a tree trying to grow tall and strong without any light and while crowded by other, taller trees.

You may wonder why there is no mention here of the effects of a lack of care and attention. This is mainly because, for any parent committed enough to be reading this book, that is unlikely to be an issue. It is also worth pointing out, though, that a child can be micro-managed while at the same time also be lacking love and nurture. Excessive scrutiny and a lack of care and attention are not two ends of the same spectrum. Super-scrutiny is not just an abundance of quality care and attention. It is the wrong kind of care and attention.

WHAT CAN WE DO TO HELP?

The tendency for a parent to micro-manage usually stems from their own anxiety. As a parent, it can be helpful to reflect on the following questions:

- Is there an area of your child's life where you have a tendency to micro-manage her?

- If your child is old enough, can you ask her what her answer to this question would be?

If you are still none the wiser, ask yourself if there is something your child does or does not do (e.g. skip meals, not take care over homework, over-exercise) that is most likely to make you jolt internally or fly off the handle.

Having identified your 'trigger area', now go on to ask yourself the following questions. Let's say, for the sake of example, your trigger is your thirteen-year-old daughter's messiness. No parent would find this easy but it really stresses you out, and leads you to nag her all the time about clearing things up.

- What feelings does it trigger in you when things are not ordered and tidy?

- What went on in your own childhood connected with tidiness and chaos?

- Do you worry that your child will turn into an adult who cannot keep life together? (Probably she will not: her thirteen-year-old self will not be her 30-year-old self.)

- Does your nagging her and getting stressed about it change your child's behaviour? (Probable answer: no! It most likely makes her tune out to your imploring and embeds the behaviour further.)

- Is your micro-managing improving your connection with your child? (Probable answer: no!)

- Does it really matter if things are a bit messy for a while? (Definite answer: no!)

SUPER-SCRUTINY

Helen's daughter, Kate, had never been a great eater. She liked to graze, was picky and ate at a snail's pace. From the age of three onwards, meal-times had often been fraught as Helen made Kate sit until everything was finished and tended to fly off the handle when she saw her pushing the food around her plate. She got cross when she found Kate's food left in her lunchbox after school, and tended to always be pushing her to eat more.

By the time Kate was ten, both she and Helen had come to somewhat dread mealtimes. When Helen asked herself the questions above, she came to realise that she had a profound anxiety that Kate might develop an eating disorder. Helen had grown up with an anorexic mother and her deepest fear was to have a child with the same issue. Over time, Helen realised that her micro-management of Kate's eating habits was actually very little to do with Kate, and all to do with her unexplored feelings from her childhood.

She worked with a therapist to explore these feelings. Over time, she stopped reacting if Kate did not eat much at a particular meal and no longer asked her all the time what she had eaten or whether she was hungry. In time, Kate began to enjoy her food more and became more open to trying new foods. Mealtimes more often became times to enjoy connecting with one another.

Pressure and expectation

Parents generally want their children to do well in life. However, there is a fine line between hoping for the best and exerting pressure. Children breathe in pressure as if it is air. They will sense it in a parent's tone of voice, look or demeanour, even when it is not verbalised. If a parent has particular expectations of a child, you can guarantee the child will know it, even when the parent believes they are doing a great job of not showing it. Whenever a parent has an inflated, rather than realistic, expectation of what a child can achieve, it almost invariably detracts from the child's mental/emotional health. It also strains the relationship, which further impacts the child's mental/emotional health.

A child responds to pressure and expectation in her own way, largely depending on her Element type. A *yin* response might be to 'give up', as she feels nothing she does is ever good enough. This can be a trigger for depression. A *yang* response might be to try harder and harder, which might be a trigger for anxiety.

Seeing the wood for the trees

▶ Focusing on their own mental/emotional health is one of the most impactful things a parent can do to help their child.

▶ What happens to one member of a family can affect all the members. Children are often the lightning rod for the whole family.

▶ The nuanced ways in which parents and children interact can have an impact on the child's mental/emotional health. Understanding the different Element types of the family members is one of the most useful ways to smooth family interactions.

▶ Super-scrutiny, over-attentiveness and micro-management of a child all increase the risk of the child becoming anxious and/or depressed.

Endnotes

1   L. Yousheng (2014) *Let the Radiant Yang Shine Forth: Lectures on Virtue*, translated by L. Zuozhi and S. Wilms (Corbett, OR: Happy Goat Productions), p. 67.

2   S. Grosz (2014) *The Examined Life: How We Lose and Find Ourselves* (London: Vintage), p. 140.

• Chapter 11 •

Times of Change

The big picture

There are times during childhood when life ticks along in a relatively smooth way. There are also times that are more turbulent and challenging. This may be due to an internal process such as an intense growth spurt, or an external event such as parents getting divorced. It may be due to a one-off traumatic event, or a protracted period when the child is under strain. During these times, a child is more vulnerable. Her *qi* is more likely to be knocked off-kilter. Therefore, she will need special care during these times to ensure that she is able to return to a place of balance.

On the one hand, times of change can be an opportunity. If circumstances are favourable, and the wind is in the right direction, a child can come through such a time in a healthier state than before. These are times when physical symptoms or emotional states that have plagued the child for years can finally be thrown off.

On the other hand, times of change are also potentially times of crisis. If a child's external circumstances are not favourable, or if she is not cared for in the right way, she may come through to the other side in worse shape than she went into such times. Pre-existing physical symptoms or emotional states may become entrenched, and new ones may develop.

It is common to trace the seeds of a mental/emotional difficulty back to a time when life was difficult, even if the problem does not show itself until later. This chapter looks at what, from a Chinese medicine perspective, happens during these times and what kind of care a child most needs to come through them as well as possible.

I have chosen here to include sections on pregnancy and birth. This may seem strange, given that nothing can be done retrospectively. I have done this in the hope that readers might impart this information to anyone who may have children in the future. Or maybe the reader will have more children. From the Chinese medicine perspective, laying down good foundations of mental/emotional health begins not even from the first day of life, but from the moment of conception.

I include this information somewhat reluctantly, however, knowing that some mothers may read it, and wish that things during their pregnancy and/or birth had been different. They may even berate themselves for not having done better. To these women, I would like to reach out and give them a big hug and encourage them to let go of their misplaced feelings of guilt. All any of us can ever do is our best, often in imperfect circumstances.

There are aspects of life over which we have no control that impact pregnancies and births. Even if our children's lives were perfect (if such a notion exists) we would not be doing them any favours by protecting them from encountering any challenges at all. Children build resilience when life, even if in the womb, during or immediately after birth, is not quite ideal.

Pregnancy

Chinese medicine has a profound understanding that whatever happens to and within a woman during pregnancy has an impact on her unborn child. It even has a specific branch called *taijiao*, which is usually translated as 'foetal education'. This discusses the impact on the foetus of a woman's life during pregnancy. In the West, it is difficult to talk about this concept without burdening pregnant women with an even greater sense of responsibility than most already feel.

Traditionally in China, *taijiao* meant that pregnant women received a lot of support from extended family. Sadly, few women in the West are afforded the same level of care and support, and most are expected to continue life as normal. Again, it feels important to discuss this topic in the hope that, if it slowly filters out to the wider community, it might change the way society treats pregnant women.

The key aspects of a woman's life that are understood to impact the foetus are:

- the rhythm of her daily life

- her diet

- her emotional state.

The last of these factors, the pregnant woman's emotional state, is the one that is most relevant in our discussion of anxiety and depression. If a woman has heightened emotions during pregnancy, it is understood to negatively impact the *shen* of the unborn child. Sun Simiao wrote:

> The most important thing for a pregnant woman's psyche is to always have a peaceful state of mind. If her heart and mind are not peaceful it brings harm to her body and is harmful for the foetus. The harm brought by anxiety is the greatest.[1]

As mother and baby are considered to be one energetic unit, if the mother's *shen* is agitated, the baby's *shen* will be agitated. Pregnancy can be a stressful time for a woman, for many different reasons. However, the more steps a woman is able to take to look after her own mental/emotional health during pregnancy, the greater the benefit to the baby.

Birth

The English comedian John Cleese wrote that 'Being born brings about a distinct change in one's lifestyle, doesn't it?'[2] In Chinese medicine, birth is considered to be a form of shock. A birth that is fraught with difficulty, full of medical intervention and traumatic to the mother obviously causes a greater degree of shock than a straightforward delivery. Nevertheless, all birth can be considered to some degree a shock, purely because of the enormity of the transition from being in the womb to being in the world. Signs that a baby is struggling with this transition are that she:

- is unsettled

- is hard to soothe

- doesn't like being put down

- sleeps in short bursts

- easily startles

- reacts strongly to the external world.

Caring for a baby who is unsettled and not sleeping well puts strain on the mother–baby relationship. The mother may have a feeling that she is doing something wrong or is somehow inadequate. It is fair to say that the first weeks and months of a baby's life are rarely straightforward, either for the baby or for those caring for her. It is important to recognise that the seeds of childhood anxiety and depression can be sown during this time.

If a mother experiences her baby as being 'difficult', it will make it harder for her to give her what she needs. It will also make it harder for mother and baby to connect. As we have already said, connection is a protective factor against childhood anxiety and depression. It is never too early to prioritise the need for connection in a baby's life.

WHAT CAN WE DO TO HELP?

Thankfully, it is relatively straightforward to soothe a baby who is struggling to adapt to being in the world. Many of the things listed below are what a parent would naturally do anyway. However, it was not that long ago that it would have been considered inconsequential whether these things happened to a baby or not. It is worth stressing here that these basic principles really do have a positive impact on a newborn baby's *qi* and *shen*, thereby increasing the chances of strong mental/emotional well-being in the future.

- Keep the umbilical cord intact until it has stopped pulsating (known as 'delayed cord clamping').

- Skin-to-skin contact as soon as possible after birth.

- Regular skin-to-skin contact in the first weeks and months of life.

- Keeping the home environment as calm and peaceful as possible.

- Carrying the baby in a sling whenever possible.

- Safe co-sleeping.

- Making sure the mother gets as much support as possible.[3]

Shock and trauma

Chinese medicine understands that shock or trauma has a particularly strong impact on the *shen* of a baby or child. As we saw in Chapter 8, it disturbs the balance between the Fire and Water Elements. If a child's Fire–Water axis has been damaged by shock or trauma, it is the mental/emotional equivalent of walking barefoot on a beach with cuts on the soles of your feet. Every time you step on a shell or a stone, the cuts will open again. It will mean that the child will go through life feeling raw and her emotional responses to events will be exaggerated. Or she may disconnect from her emotions and become cut off as a way of avoiding the pain. She will be more easily knocked off-kilter by what life throws at her. It will be difficult for her to come back to a contented and harmonious state.

The Fire–Water axis can also be understood as the fundamental balance between *yang* (Fire) and *yin* (Water). When the balance between these two Elements is impaired, it often leads to an excess of *yang* and a depletion of *yin*. Or, to put it another way, Fire begins to rage and there is insufficient Water to control it. The mental/emotional manifestation of this is anxiety. The child feels constantly on edge because *yin* is insufficient to create an internal sense of calm. At times, this tips over into more extreme panic or emotional meltdown, when the excess *yang* agitates the *shen*. The Chinese texts describe this feeling as the sensation of a drum beating away at the heart, causing a kind of pounding sensation.

There are certain events or situations that would be experienced by almost every child as a kind of trauma, for example physical or sexual abuse, or the loss of a parent. However, it is helpful to understand trauma not as an event but as a response. Depending on her innate constitution, each child will have a unique emotional response to a particular event. For one child, having a mother who is away a lot might be deeply distressing, whereas another child might take it in her stride. The cumulative effect of lots of small events may also amount to a kind of shock.

A child's emotional response to life events will be determined in part by the sensitivity of her *shen* and in part by her Five Element constitutional nature. It is unhelpful to assume a particular response and more helpful to observe, with an open mind, whatever response an individual child has to a particular event.

Although Chinese medical texts stress the importance of protecting young children from the vagaries of life, it is simply not possible for parents and carers to always protect a child from something she might experience as traumatic. When a child has felt shocked by something, there are various measures that can be taken to help lessen the impact.

WHAT CAN WE DO TO HELP?

- Safe and loving physical touch from trusted caregivers after a child has had a difficult experience helps the child's *qi* to become regulated again. Depending on the degree of trauma, touch is beneficial not only in the immediate aftermath but in the longer term.

- Ensuring rhythm and consistency in a child's daily life also helps to create a feeling of safety after a time of strain or difficulty.

- Time spent in nature can soothe the child's nervous system when it has become jangled.

- Opportunities for sleep and rest help a child to regain her equilibrium after a traumatic experience.

- For an older child, allowing her to talk about a difficult experience (if and when she wants to) encourages her *qi* to begin to regulate again. She needs an adult to bear witness to her feelings and listen without judgement, rather than any particular verbal response. Sometimes, it is better for this to happen with somebody other than a parent. A child may sense that what she says might induce strong emotions in her parent and this might impede her from freely expressing her emotions.

Big growth spurts and developmental leaps

A child does not tend to grow at a steady pace, but has phases where growth slackens and phases where it accelerates. A child grows at her fastest during the first year of life and during adolescence. It is astonishing to think that a baby arrives in the world totally unable to look after any of her own needs and yet by the end of the first year will have begun to move, feed herself and communicate verbally.

Every time of accelerated physical growth and every development milestone is fuelled by *qi, yang* and *essence*. We tend to forget that growing is a tiring process. A useful analogy is that of a duck who glides along the surface of the water with apparently no effort, but underneath is paddling hard. Growth and development are the same: seemingly effortless but actually requiring an immense amount of hard work and energy.

If a child's life is such that her resources of *qi* are all going to meet the demands that she is under, then her process of growth and development is going to become impaired. For example, if she finds the school day, academic demands, extracurricular activities and social interaction tiring, her internal resources will be used up trying to manage her daily life and there will not be sufficient left over for growth and development. Instead of *qi, yin, yang, blood* and *essence* building strong foundations of both physical and mental/emotional health, they are being diverted to meet external demands. It is rather like spending everything you earn, rather than putting some into a savings account. This might be fine for a period of time but when you have an extra, unforeseen expense you find you do not have the resources to cope.

For a child, when she hits an accelerated growth phase, her resources may not be sufficient to fuel it. This is when imbalance arises, and this imbalance may manifest in either a physical symptom or, as is frequently the case, a mental/emotional symptom, such as anxiety or depression.

There is a popular Chinese tale about a sprout farmer, who was so keen for his sprouts to grow quickly that he pulled them up out of the ground in order to try to make them grow taller and faster. To his shock and horror, he woke one morning to find they had all died. Instead of concentrating on giving them the nourishment they needed and trusting them to grow in their own time, he forced the process. This is often used as a cautionary tale of how *not* to care for children. Unlike the farmer, we need to trust that children will grow and develop in their own time and at their own pace.

Luke began becoming increasingly anxious around the age of thirteen. Not only did he feel anxious, but his behaviour was becoming more aggressive. His self-esteem was also low and he frequently talked about feeling like a failure. Luke had a busy life. He went to a school that pushed its students academically, and had a couple of hours of homework every evening. He also played two musical instruments. His parents insisted that he did half an hour of practice on each instrument every day, after school. Saturdays were taken up with playing hockey for the local club team.

Luke was beginning the huge developmental leap of adolescence when his symptoms began. His body was not only growing at an extraordinary rate, but also changing. His parents were, at first, reluctant to ease up on any of his musical or sporting activities. They felt that achieving in these areas would bolster Luke's self-esteem.

In time, they began to see that the opposite was actually the case. The strain Luke felt was contributing to his falling self-esteem, as well as his anxiety and aggressive behaviour. Together with Luke, they came to a mutual agreement that he would pause both instruments, lessons and practice, for the foreseeable future and could resume them if and when he chose at any point.

During the hour that he had spent practising each day after school, he now hung out with friends or simply came home and watched TV. This small change, alongside having some acupuncture treatment and bringing bedtime forward by half an hour, meant that within a couple of months Luke began to thrive again.

As we have said many times before, the key is to look at the capacity each child has for a busy or demanding life, and to be mindful that this might change as the child grows. When a child begins to feel anxious on a frequent basis, or when her mood appears to be lowered over a period of time, it may be simply because she cannot fuel the growth or development that is trying to take place inside her as well as manage her everyday life.

WHAT CAN WE DO TO HELP?

- If you notice that a child is in a phase of being constantly tired or more emotionally volatile than usual, consider that she may be in the midst of a growth spurt or a developmental leap. Ask what pressures can be taken off her, to free up some of her *qi* to support her internal processes.

- It is even more important during these times that the child gets sufficient sleep and eats well. She is less likely to get away with skimping on these fundamental pillars of health than she might at other times.

- Big growth spurts and developmental leaps involve a surge of *yang*. Ensure that the *yin* aspects of life (such as downtime, time at home, time with family, as discussed in Chapter 12) are present to help stabilise the child.

Illness/fevers

Illnesses, particularly those that involve fever, are also considered in Chinese medicine to be times of volatility and change. Sun Simiao described fevers as 'transformations and steamings', the implication being that through the process of having a fever, a child 'transforms' in some way. He said that 'when the major and minor steamings are all finished, the baby has become a human being.'[4]

This view is backed up by parents who often report that, after an illness, their child made a leap in terms of her speech or maturity, for example, or that she began sleeping properly for the first time, or her appetite increased.

So, from the Chinese medicine perspective, fevers are considered an important stage of development and a vital part of the maturation process. The important point, however, is not so much whether a child gets a fever but how she is cared for throughout.

While they can be opportunities, fevers and illnesses are also vulnerable times in a child's life. If a child gets a particularly bad illness, or does not have appropriate care through a mild illness, she may come out the other side in a place of less equilibrium than she went into it. As the body and the mind are one unit, even a purely physical illness may leave a child with a mental/emotional imbalance. This process can be explained by the Chinese medicine concept of a 'lingering pathogenic factor'.

Lingering pathogens

When a child gets a bacterial or viral infection, her *qi* will mobilise to fight off the infection. It is the battle that ensues between what is known as 'upright *qi*' and 'evil *qi*' (i.e. the bacteria or virus) that often creates the symptoms during the acute stage of an illness. Afterwards, once the 'upright *qi*' has won the battle, the child may need time to recuperate but, ideally, the pathogen has been successfully fought off and will have left the child's body.

However, what often happens is a little different. The child ostensibly gets better from an illness, but instead of entirely throwing off the pathogen, a latent form of it lingers around afterwards. An example of this is glandular fever. A minority of sufferers get over the acute symptoms of the virus but find they have other, usually milder, symptoms for a long time afterwards.

A famous Chinese doctor, Dr Shen, had a wonderful analogy for this. He said that if a burglar comes to your house in the middle of the night, you have two choices. You can either fight him and (hopefully) win and throw him out of the house. Or, you can shoot him dead. The immediate problem is over but you are left with a dead body in your house, which will cause longer-term problems. Both these outcomes are possible when a child gets an acute illness.

The second scenario (i.e. the burglar being shot dead in the house) is most likely to occur if the child does not get sufficient rest and care throughout the acute stage of the illness. The use of antibiotics (while sometimes necessary) also increases the chance of this outcome. Parents often report that a child has 'not been herself' or has stopped sleeping well or developed a chronic cough, for example, ever since a particular illness. This is a sure sign that she has been left with a lingering pathogen. The burglar is dead on the floor, as it were.

Lingering pathogens may have a long-lasting impact on the mental/emotional health of a child. They disturb the flow of *qi*. This can create a tendency for a particular emotion to become the child's habitual state. Lingering pathogens also consume *qi*. They place a strain on the child, as if she constantly has a heavy rucksack on her back. The strain this causes often leads to a deficiency in one or more of the Vital Substances. One manifestation of this is a mental/emotional imbalance.

Thankfully, there is a lot that can be done to ensure that a child comes through an acute illness without a lingering pathogen.

WHAT CAN WE DO TO HELP?

- Despite what the cold and flu remedy adverts would have us believe, life should not carry on as normal through acute illness. A child needs to gather her resources to fight the illness, not use them to fulfil her usual daily schedule. It is vital that a child stops her usual life when she is ill, stays at home and rests.

- Chinese medicine understands that a child needs a day of recuperation for every day of an illness. So if she had a chest infection that lasted four days, she should have four days more in which to recover her *qi*. This means four days with lots of rest, low stimulation, nourishing food and lots of nurture. There is huge pressure from schools for children to attend even when they are in the throes of an illness and definitely as soon as they are over the worst of it. It can also be difficult for parents who struggle to get the time off work to care for sick children. However, it is very short-sighted of us as a society to think this way. Short-term sacrifice can have huge long-term benefits in the form of healthier children.

- A child is less likely to develop a lingering pathogen if she is cared for one on one by a familiar and trusted adult through an acute illness. A child does not yet have a reservoir of *qi* she can dig into when she is ill, because she is using all of it purely to grow and develop. Therefore, she will 'feed' off the *qi* of her main caregiver in order to get through the illness. This is why parents often say they feel exhausted when they have been sitting at home looking after a poorly child.

- While of course there is a place for antibiotics, their use increases the chance of a child coming through an illness with a lingering pathogen. When antibiotics are necessary, a few sessions of acupuncture treatment can help to bring a child's *qi* back to a place of equilibrium and expel any lingering pathogens.

Adolescence

Adolescence is a time of transformation. It is also the one that takes a child much closer to adulthood. It is characterised by enormous flux, as if the child's entire mind and body are recalibrating. In Chinese medicine terms, several things are going on:

- The physical and psychological changes that take place during adolescence are fuelled by a surge of *yang*. *Yang* fuels the rapid physical growth, the bodily changes and the reaching for independence that characterise this time. So there tends to be more *heat* around in the body during the adolescent years.

- The Water Element is under strain during adolescence because it is the source of *yang* which fuels the rapid growth and development.

- *Qi* is prone to stagnating during adolescence. As well as a general impatience to be earning money, drinking, driving, etc., this is because the drive for independence is often greater than the degree of independence a teen is given. The mismatch between the two creates strong feelings of constraint, which have the effect of stagnating *qi*. This explains the characteristic moodiness of many teenagers, moodiness being a key symptom of *qi* stagnation.

- The Earth Element is under strain during adolescence. Teenagers often consume huge amounts of food to fuel their rapid growth, as well as having to work harder than before. Both these things strain the *qi* of the Earth Element.

With all this change taking place, a teen is vulnerable to imbalances settling in. The balance of *qi*, *yin*, *yang*, *shen* and *blood* are all thrown up into the air. If a teen is unhappy, stressed, tired or a combination of all three, they are less likely to land back down in a balanced fashion. It is also a common time for a teen to begin feeling anxious. This is because the surge of *yang* mentioned above inflames and magnifies feelings that may have been going on beforehand at a low level, but are now brought into focus.

WHAT CAN WE DO TO HELP?

If you have a teen in mind who is struggling, ask yourself the following questions:

- Does she have enough *yin* aspects to her daily life, such as sleep, rest, downtime, time with the family? (See Chapter 12)

- Does the teen feel constrained by the level of freedom and independence she is allowed? Are there areas where she could safely be allowed more?

- Is she feeling connected, to both family and friends? Remaining connected with teens can be difficult for parents. But connection (see Chapter 9) is of paramount importance through the teenage years. This includes ongoing connection with family but also new and increasingly important connection with friends.

Times of stress and strain

In the words of the poet Henry Longfellow, in the poem 'The Rainy Day', 'into each life some rain must fall'. It is a rare child who makes it through to adulthood without some degree of adversity. This is also no bad thing, as it is adversity that builds resilience. The *shen* of a child is steeled by experiencing difficulty, as long as the right kind of support is provided and as long as the degree of difficulty is not too great for the *shen* of that particular child to manage.

However, the seeds of anxiety and depression are also most likely to take root during times of adversity. The parents of children who come to my clinic frequently say that they first noticed a change in their child when, for example, she had friendship difficulties at school, she lost her grandmother, the family moved towns or a sibling was very ill. It is during these phases of change or difficulty that imbalances in *qi* are most likely to arise. Therefore, these are the times when the principles and ideas laid out in this book become most important. These are the times when a child is at her most vulnerable, and consequently when she is most in need of attuned care and appropriate nurture.

Chinese medicine has a branch called *yang sheng* which roughly translates as 'nurturing life'. It understands that prevention is more important than cure. At its core is the philosophy that how we live our lives, alongside constitution, is the biggest determining factor in both our physical and mental/emotional health. If a child is supported to incorporate the principles discussed in this book, she is more likely to continue living by them during tough times. It is much harder to adopt new habits during periods of stress than it is to carry on doing what we are used to. If a child is shown how to 'nurture life' as she grows up, she is more likely to be able to keep doing the same when times are difficult.

There are no new pieces of advice to give about how to support a child's mental/emotional health during times of stress and strain. Everything discussed so far just becomes more important. Engendering good connections, having a balanced daily life, getting enough sleep, eating well, doing appropriate exercise: all help to support and protect the balance of *qi* in a child under strain.

Seeing the wood for the trees

▶ The foundations of a child's mental/emotional health begin to be laid down during pregnancy. The mother's emotional state impacts the *qi* and *shen* of the foetus.

▶ A baby's transition from womb to world is, in itself, a kind of shock, and everything should be done to cushion the process for the baby.

▶ During childhood, there are many times of change and transformation, which can be either a crisis or an opportunity. A child needs extra care during these times.

▶ If a child has appropriate care during a time of change, it lessens the chances of anxiety and/or depression emerging.

▶ Key times of change, during which a child is more susceptible to developing an imbalance or disharmony, are: shock and trauma, big growth spurts and developmental leaps, illnesses and fevers, adolescence, and times of stress and strain.

Endnotes

1   Quoted in P. Deadman (2014) 'Taijiao (foetal education)', *Journal of Chinese Medicine* 106: 48–54, p. 49.

2   R. Skynner and J. Cleese (1997) *Families and How to Survive Them* (London: Vermilion), p. 95.

3   In China, there is a concept known as 'doing the month'. This involves the mother resting and the other members of the household taking over domestic duties. It is understood to be important so that the mother can recoup her energy after pregnancy and birth.

4   S. Wilms (trans.) (2013) *Venerating the Root: Part 1*. Sun Simiao's *Bei Ji Qian Jin Yao Fang*, Volume 5: Paediatrics (Corbett, OR: Happy Goat Productions), p. 15.

• Chapter 12 •

The *Yin* and *Yang* of Daily Life

The big picture

The rhythm, pace and value of our daily activities play a big part in determining how we feel, because feelings tend to follow behaviour. Young children have very little say in their daily routines. It would of course often lead to disaster to give children complete responsibility for how they fill their days. However, there is no doubt that the daily lives of some children are making them sick. More specifically, they are causing some children to become anxious and depressed.

There are two defining characteristics of children that we need to bear in mind when thinking about the impact their daily life has on them. These are:

- Children are constantly growing and developing. The implications of this fact are often overlooked. It means that a proportion of a child's *qi* needs to be available to support the process of growth and development. If a child's life is too demanding, there will not be enough *qi* available for this process.

- Children are inherently *yang* in nature. This means that the nature of their daily life needs to be *yin*, in order to provide a balance to their *yang*. We will look at what this means later.

If you are caring for older children, you might want to skip the sections 'From the womb to the world' and '*Yin*-building: the toddler years and early childhood', and go straight to 'Middle childhood and the teenage years: avoiding storms of *yang*'.

From the womb to the world

Humans are born at an earlier stage in their development than other mammals. Therefore, the first nine months of life are sometimes referred to as a 'second pregnancy'. Babies require a womb-like environment in the first months of life in order to complete their development, more of which is done outside the womb than in other mammals.

The early Chinese medicine texts on paediatrics contain many references to the importance of shielding a baby from anything sudden, loud or unfamiliar. For example, Sun Simiao urged parents to:

> Constantly beware of fright while rearing small children. Do not let them hear loud noises and, when holding them in your arms, be still and gentle. Do not let them be frightened or startled. Moreover, when there is thunder in the sky, plug the children's ears and at the same time make some other subtle noises in order to distract them.[1]

A young baby may experience, for example, a sudden noise or a stranger picking him up as a kind of micro-shock. He is so *yang* in nature at this time of life that it does not take much to agitate or disturb him. Of course, it is impossible to always shield a baby from anything that he might find disturbing. As long as he is soothed back to a state of equilibrium, this rarely has any long-term consequences.

However, if a baby is constantly exposed to micro-shocks, they may agitate his nervous system and disturb his *shen*. This may mean that, as he grows up, he becomes hypersensitive to his environment. He has an exaggerated response to stimuli. This will predispose him to feeling anxious, unsettled and agitated.

Ben started nursery when he was nine months old, when his mother had to return to work. Although he seemed happy to go there, he would come home at the end of the day quite agitated. His mum noticed that it would not take much to reduce him to tears, he took longer to get to sleep, and he was having many more meltdowns. After three months, things were no better and his mum started to explore other childcare options. She found a local childminder, who had just two other children to look after. Almost immediately, Ben became more settled. The meltdowns stopped, his sleep improved and he became much calmer.

As always, it is important to remember that the key factor is always the interaction between a baby and his environment. A baby with strong *shen* and very robust *qi* will be less sensitive to his environment than one with a more delicate *shen*.

WHAT CAN WE DO TO HELP?

- Most babies will thrive from having a protected, nurturing environment.

- When a baby does become agitated, explore what helps him to regain his equilibrium. It might be something as simple as being held, rocked or sung to.

- If a baby seems to be frequently agitated and unsettled, identify what it is in his environment that is causing this. For example, it might be that there is too much noise, too many different people or too much heightened emotion.

Yin-building: the toddler years and early childhood

Depending on the child, somewhere in the second or third year of life, he will become more able to withstand the unpredictable nature of the external environment. He is still, however, very *yang* in nature and therefore needs many aspects of his environment to be *yin*. These aspects may include:

Repetition

For most adults, reading the same story every night would be the epitome of boring. The reason children love it is because any sort of repetition is *yin* in nature and therefore helps to counterbalance their predominance of *yang*. In turn, it helps them to feel safe and secure.

Toddlers and young children tend to enjoy watching the same thing on television, going to the same playground and playing the same games. It's helpful to know there is a reason for this, rather than it just being a random quirk. It is helping to build the child's foundations of *yin*, which will provide a good foundation for future mental and physical health.

Rhythm

Having a rhythm to daily life is also *yin*-building. Getting up, eating meals, having naps and going to bed at roughly the same time each day helps to nurture a child's *yin* and create security. This does not mean creating a rigid routine. It is to do with life having a steady rhythm to it, which is comforting, like the tick of a clock or the beat of a song.

Parents sometimes worry that if their child is used to a certain rhythm, it will mean he will not be able to adapt or cope when something changes, for example, on holiday or when he goes to stay with his grandparents. They worry they are creating a rod for their own back. From the Chinese medicine perspective, the opposite is true. Having a steady rhythm to life in the early years is *yin*-building, which means a child is better able to be flexible and adaptable when he grows. Remember that *yin* is soft and supple and therefore helps a child to adapt in order to find his way past an obstacle when one arises. As Lao Tzu said in the *Tao Te Ching*, 'the tree that bends doesn't break in the wind'.

Nurture

The right kind of nurture helps to build a child's reserves of *yin*. This is another area where a parent may worry that they are creating problems for the future if they always respond to their child's needs. They may be concerned that if they comfort a child every time he cries, sit beside him when he is ill and help him to go to sleep at night that he will never learn to do these things himself.

However, giving a child nurture does not just help him in that moment. It is also a way of imparting the ability for him to do the same for himself when he is older. Children who get what they need in the early years of life have a much higher chance of growing up to be emotionally balanced adults than those who do not.

A psychologist called Harry Harlow did some fascinating, if ethically dubious, research with monkeys to look at the impact mothering had on their ability to move into independence. He put them into four groups. One group were kept in cages with their mothers, one group had no mothers, a third were in cages with wire frames shaped like a mother, and the fourth were in cages with a piece of furry cloth shaped like a mother.

He noticed that the group put with their mothers would happily go off and explore and then come back to their mother, and then go off and explore again. The group without any kind of mother did not play or explore and grew up unable to cope with social situations.

The group with the wire-frame mothers acted in a similar way to those without any mother figure at all. The group with the furry cloth shaped like mothers did not do as well as the group who had their real mothers but did a lot better than the group with the wire mothers.

He concluded that the group with their mothers, and to some degree even the ones with the cloth mothers, were given the chance to steady themselves after going off and exploring. The purpose of the mother was to help calm their anxiety that came from having new experiences.

However, even with nurture the idea of balance is important. As well as giving a child the nurture he needs, the job of a parent is also to instil in him the confidence that he can cope with the world as he grows older. In Chapter 3, we discussed the idea of aiming for a balance between protection and exposure. As they grow, children need to be exposed to some of the difficulties of life to develop an inner confidence in their ability to cope with them and learn from them.

Peace and quiet

Too much noise and hubbub is *yang* in nature and therefore can agitate a young child and hamper his ability to build his *yin*. More specifically, in Chinese medicine terms, it agitates the *qi* of the Water and Wood Elements, and has a depleting effect on *yin*. Times of quiet and stillness are crucial components of a young child's life.

When Maeve started school, at the age of four, she soon began taking herself off to the corner of the classroom and sitting with her hands over her ears. Being a particularly sensitive child, she found the noise and hubbub of the classroom too intense and stimulating. Her parents decided to homeschool her for a couple of years.

She started school again when she was seven, by which time she found it much easier. She still occasionally needed some time out in a quiet room, which thankfully her school was able to provide. Most of the time she managed being in the classroom very well. Having a few years at home gave her *yin* more time to become replete.

Middle childhood and the teenage years: avoiding storms of *yang*

From the age of about seven or eight, if the previous years have been conducive to their development, a child will have a more solid foundation of *yin*. However, *yin* does not reach its peak until much later, in the teenage years when a child stops growing. So, although an older child does not need such an extremely *yin* environment to be able to thrive, a daily life which is too *yang* may still be detrimental.

The nature of many older children's lives does not enable their mental/ emotional health to thrive. The aspects of life which we will now discuss are too *yang* and agitate the *shen*. As always, every child has a different tolerance to all these things. In each case, the aim is to create a daily life that is manageable. One child may cope well with lots of intellectual stimulation and academic pressure; for another, it may be a factor that pushes him towards feeling anxious or depressed.

Over-scheduling

The more hectic a child's daily schedule, the more depleting it is to his *yin*. When *yin* declines, *yang* naturally rises. This means that a child may spend his life in an almost constant 'buzz', rarely ever truly feeling calm or relaxed. His schedule might mean he goes from one activity to another, squeezing in mealtimes along the way, before being hurried into bed at night, and then starting all over again the next day.

As Lao Tzu wrote in the *Tao Te Ching*, 'nature does not hurry, yet everything is accomplished'. Sometimes, anxious feelings are the mind making a plea not to be continuously and exhaustingly overstimulated. It is not necessarily psychologically healthy for a child to do as much as may be physically possible.

Our sense of what is normal, in terms of a child's schedule, has arguably become quite skewed. Many people do not blink an eyelid at a nine-year-old who goes to school, has an extracurricular activity each day after school, and several more at the weekend too. On top of this, he may need to fit in music practice, homework, birthday parties and several hours on his games console. Mealtimes become something that have to be squeezed in between activities and he gets into bed at night either so exhausted he is asleep before his head hits the pillow or so overstimulated that he cannot sleep.

This kind of 'extreme *yang*' schedule is, for the vast majority of children, not sustainable. Some price is paid somewhere down the line, even if the child appears to be able to handle it in the short term. It means that much of the child's *qi* is consumed by meeting the demands of his lifestyle. His mental/emotional development may suffer as a result. Feelings of anxiety and/or depression may be a signal that his lifestyle is simply not one that allows him to be content and happy. Amidst all this activity, his emerging nature, governed by his *shen*, has become lost and he becomes disconnected from his true self and purpose.

Screen time

Screens have become an integral part of the lives of older children and teens. They have created tremendous opportunities and, in many ways, enhanced the lives of young people. For example, during the lockdowns imposed in many parts of the world during the pandemic of 2020–2021, the only way many children were able to stay connected with their friends was via digital technology.

How long?

However, if you sense a 'but' coming, you are right. Good mental/emotional health arises out of a balanced life. Too much of almost anything is detrimental, and screens are no exception. It is common for children today to spend the vast majority of their waking hours when they are not at school (and sometimes when they are at school) on one type of digital device or another.

Asking how long a child can spend on a screen without it negatively impacting her is like asking how long a piece of string is. I know of children who spend eight to ten hours a day (when not at school) on a device of one kind or another but whose mental/emotional health is good. I know of other children whose anxiety spikes after just 30 minutes on a screen. The answer is not to look at the clock but to look at the child.

What?

How long a child spends on his devices may be a source of concern, but what he does on them is of greater importance. Inanely scrolling through Instagram for hours is very different to intentionally looking for specific information or chatting to a friend. When being on a device distracts a child from something that gives her purpose or raises her spirit, it has a negative impact on her *shen*. When her screen-time activities further her sense of purpose or her connections, they can boost her mental/emotional health.

Why?

Equally relevant is also the question of why a child is on a phone or tablet. We have alluded several times already to the importance of looking at what is driving behaviour, and being on a device is no different. Some common reasons a child may escape into the online world are:

- Losing himself in the online world is more appealing or less anxiety-inducing than real life.

- He has become so used to external validation that unless he is constantly connected, he does not feel good about himself.

- He is running away from his feelings. Being on his phone means he does not have to connect or sit with emotions he finds uncomfortable.

- He is so used to being overstimulated that he fears a comedown if he disconnects.

- He is bored, and picking up a device is an easy solution.

The impact of screen time on a child's *qi*

In my paediatric acupuncture clinic, I have seen some very specific effects on children of their spending large amounts of time on screens.

EXCESSIVE SCREEN TIME AGITATES LIVER *QI*

The eyes are the sensory orifice connected with the Liver. The fast-moving images and hypervisual stimulation of many video games agitate the Liver *qi* via the eyes. Most screen-time activities also involve being stationary. Liver *qi* has a particular need for movement in order to maintain its balance. Long periods in front of screens frequently lead to *qi* stagnation. This is one of the most commonly seen pathologies in children who are depressed.

EXCESSIVE TIME PLAYING VIDEO GAMES DISTURBS THE KIDNEYS

Many video games are intensely competitive and cause children to become adrenalised. When a child becomes grumpy when he has to stop playing them, it is because he is going through an adrenaline withdrawal.

In Chinese medicine terms, whenever a child is adrenalised, he is digging into the reserves of Kidney *yin*. As we have seen, childhood should be all about building up reserves of *yin*, not depleting them. *Yin* deficiency is often an underlying imbalance in a child who is anxious.

EXCESSIVE TIME SPENT ON SOCIAL MEDIA DISTURBS THE HEART AND THE *SHEN*

Social media is often a contributory factor to the poor mental/emotional well-being of children who come to my clinic, especially girls. Adolescence, in particular, is a time of heightened self-consciousness, which is now lived out under the scrutiny of so-called 'friends' on platforms such as Instagram, Snapchat and TikTok.

A child, when he is on his phone, is often on a constant emotional roller coaster depending on whether he is 'liked', 'friended', 'unfriended', included or excluded. He is also often being barraged with images of others who are, apparently, living the perfect life and against whom he falls into comparing himself. A child needs to develop an internal sense that he is 'OK', accepted for who he is, and loved.

In order for the *shen* to be calm and the Heart to be peaceful, a child needs downtime and periods when he is not stimulated. Today, downtime is often synonymous with time flicking through social media on a phone which would arguably be better described as 'uptime'.

The last word on screens

Connection, which was the subject of Chapter 9, is more important to a child's mental/emotional health than anything else. Despite all the pitfalls of screen time, it is also important to point out that the drive behind it for many kids is to connect with others. If battles over screens have the result that the connection between parent and child becomes diminished, then getting a child off her phone may be a pyrrhic victory for the parent.

Once again, the key is to look at the child and see how screen time is affecting her as an individual, and how it fits into the balance of her life.

WHAT CAN WE DO TO HELP?

- Before assuming that a child's screen time is detrimental to her mental/emotional health, look at the individual child and reflect on whether that really is the case and, if so, what impact it is having on her. A good way to do this is to notice what happens when a child is not able to be on her phone.

- Be curious as to why the child is spending what seems like excessive time on her screen. What need is it serving?

- Put your focus on the rest of the child's life. Spending endless time on screens is a symptom, not a root cause of a problem. What is the root cause?

Too much mental stimulation

There is a strong understanding in Chinese medicine, and in Daoist thought, that excessive mental activity is not good for one's health, in particular a person's mental/emotional health. This truth applies even more strongly to children, who, because of their predominance of *yang*, have an even greater need for physical movement. Because of this, they also have a stronger propensity for *qi* to rise up to the head than adults. Mental activity does not only mean intellectual work but also encompasses the act of thinking.

Many children of school age spend the vast bulk of their time doing cerebral activities, whether it be learning at school, reading, something on a screen or simply thinking. This can lead to 'counterflow *qi*', which means that a child's *qi* gets stuck in his head and becomes 'knotted'. It is very hard to feel calm and peaceful in this state. The antidote is to do something physical, which helps to bring *qi* back down into the body and get it flowing.

So a combination of lots of mental activity and not very much physical activity can, over time, create the kind of feeling that we might get as adults when we have spent too long in front of our computer screens and feel ruffled and ill-tempered. For some children this is an almost constant state. Even though it is not pleasant, it can be hard for a child to recognise this and do something to pull herself out of it. Counterflow *qi*, over a period of time, may create anxiety.

WHAT CAN WE DO TO HELP?

With a particular child in mind, reflect on the following questions:

- Does the child have a balance of physical and mental activities throughout her day?

- Does the child have frequent opportunities for physical activity throughout her day?

- Does the child have an opportunity to run around immediately after coming out of school?

- Does an older child or teen have a break in which she moves around, after every hour that she sits at her desk studying?

Desire and craving

Closely related to thinking and mental activity is desire and craving. The first chapter of the *Su Wen* says, 'One should live a quiet life with few desires so that one can preserve one's *qi* and guard one's mind in order to avoid disease. Thus if emotions are absent and craving is curbed, the heart is peaceful and there is no fear.'[2]

Children in Western societies are growing up in an era of rampant consumerism. Advertising would have a young child believe that if he has a new phone or the latest edition of branded trainers, he will be happier. In fact, once a child has whatever item he has been craving, there is usually only a short window of time before he is no longer satisfied by that, and the desire for the next thing begins to grow in him.

Of course, the Daoist ideal of restraining craving entirely is not a realistic goal for most children. However, the degree of craving and desire that has become an accepted part of many children's lives is now a huge risk factor for mental/emotional issues. This is not only because it turns out that having a new pair of trainers does not really make the child happy. It is also because of the impact this constant state of desire has on a child. It agitates the *shen* and knots the *qi*, both of which predispose a child to then feeling anxious and/or depressed.

WHAT CAN WE DO TO HELP?

- Limit the exposure a child (especially a young one) has to advertising wherever possible. This can be done by not allowing a young child access to social media and limiting exposure to TV programmes that are interspersed with adverts.

- We adults need to set an example to children in this area. If children see us craving material things and spending much of our leisure time going shopping, they will grow up to do the same.

- We can initiate conversations with children about what makes us happy, and the difference between the short-term feeling of excitement we might get when we open a present and the long-term feeling of contentment we might get from having had a new experience or having spent time around people we love.

Seeing the wood for the trees

▶ The priority in the first year or so of life is to create an easy transition from womb to world that prioritises a protective, nurturing environment for the child.

▶ A child has a predominance of *yang* and therefore needs a lifestyle that contains lots of *yin* aspects. These include:

  – repetition

- rhythm

- nurture

- peace and quiet.

▶ A child uses a certain amount of his *qi* to support the process of growth and development. Therefore, a daily schedule that is too demanding and busy for a particular child may use up resources that should be directed at building the foundations of mental/emotional (and thus physical) health.

▶ This remains the case (although to a lesser degree as the child grows) up until the time when a child has stopped growing.

▶ Four key *yang*-activating aspects of life are:

- over-scheduling

- screen time

- mental activity

- desire/craving.

Endnotes

1   S. Wilms (trans.) (2013) *Venerating the Root: Part 1*. Sun Simiao's *Bei Ji Qian Jin Yao Fang*, Volume 5: Paediatrics (Corbett, OR: Happy Goat Productions), p. 123.

2   *The Yellow Emperor's Classic of Internal Medicine – Simple Questions (Huang Di Nei Jing Su Wen)* (1979) (Beijing: People's Health Publishing House), p. 3.

• Chapter 13 •

Exercise

The big picture

Exercise is 'a good thing'. Every traditional medicine culture, as far back as Hippocrates, recognised the importance of exercise for both physical and mental health. The Latin phrase *mens sana in corpore sano* ('a healthy mind in a healthy body') conveys the idea that physical exercise is an important part of mental and psychological well-being.

Today, exercise is often prescribed by psychologists and physicians for children who are struggling with their mental well-being. Parents all over the world see exercise as a vital way of preventing obesity, and getting their children off screens and sofas.

However, little is said about what kind of exercise might be appropriate for an individual child, and about how much exercise is required at different ages. As we have seen in other chapters, what might suit one child might hinder another. When we understand the effects that different types of exercise have on a child's *qi*, on his *blood* and *jing*, and on the balance of *yin/yang*, it helps us to take a more individualised approach.

● SORTING OUT SOME COMMON CONFUSIONS

We sometimes fail to differentiate between exercise, movement and sport. Exercise implies an activity that is carried out to improve health or fitness. Sport usually contains a competitive element. We tend not to pay much attention simply to movement for movement's sake in the West. In Chinese medicine, movement is understood as having great value in its own right, as a way of keeping the mind and body healthy.

We also often fail to understand the difference between health and fitness. We need to educate our children to understand that the goal of exercise is not only to be fit but also to improve overall health. For example, somebody might be fit enough to run a marathon but have a weak immune system, making them very fit but not very healthy.

The reason for exercising

Not so long ago, physical activity was woven into the fabric of life in a way that it is not in the modern world. Many children lead very sedentary lives, getting from A to B by car, sitting behind a desk for much of the school day and spending a lot of their leisure time on screens. As a result of this, many children do not develop the ability to sense what level and type of exercise their body needs. Rather than taking place naturally as part of daily life, physical activity often needs to be consciously timetabled into a child's life.

While, of course, one child may simply enjoy exercise, another may only do it because he is told to, another because he is trying to find an adrenaline rush, another because he feels better for pushing himself to the limit, and another because he wants to look better. For some, exercise is inextricably linked with competitive sport. In many schools, being a sporty child is a ticket to social acceptance and higher self-esteem.

While exercising for these reasons does not necessarily negate the many physical and emotional benefits, what is missing for most children is the opportunity to develop the habit of living well in the physical body. We do not teach children to become physically active purely as a way of enjoying the expression of their body. Being comfortable in his body helps a child to be comfortable in his mind. The flow of *qi* in the body affects the flow of *qi* in the mind, and vice versa. So, if we want to support a child to be mentally and emotionally contented, we need to help him to pay attention to his body as well as his thoughts and feelings.

The Chinese medicine view

Most people would list the key benefits of exercise as improving aerobic fitness, muscular strength and flexibility. Chinese medicine considers this a rather limited view of exercise. It understands that, as well as conferring these benefits, exercise can help a person become more grounded, cultivate stillness and mindfulness, and also help with breathing practices. Chinese medicine considers certain activities as exercise that, in the West, we would not classify in that way, for example, the gentle movements of *tai qi* and *qi gong*.

Ultimately, the reason why exercise of all sorts can benefit the mental/emotional well-being of a child is because of its ability to impact the flow of *qi*. As we have seen, anxiety and/or depression arise when the normal movements of *qi* have become impaired, for example, stagnant or 'knotted'. Therefore, in order to find the right exercise to benefit an individual child, we need to look at the particular way in which his flow of *qi* has become imbalanced.

Exercise in childhood

The types of exercise that most children in the West do are, from the Chinese medicine perspective, quite intensive. Anything that raises the heart rate and induces sweating consumes a considerable amount of *qi*. Strenuous exercise requires a lot of *blood* to nourish the muscles and the limbs. If these kinds of exercises (e.g. running, swimming) are done very frequently, without many days off in between, the body starts digging in to its reserves of *yin* to manage the needs of the exercise.

When a child is growing, a large proportion of his *qi* and *blood* needs to be available to support the growth process. His body is still considered a work in progress and therefore is not yet as robust as an adult body might be in terms of the degree of exercise that can be tolerated. A key Chinese medical text, *The Spiritual Pivot* (*Ling Shu*), writes that 'Children's flesh is fragile, their blood is scanty, and their *qi* is weak.'[1] Too much exercise at too young an age can therefore make a child vulnerable to physical injury. However, it can also have a negative impact on the child's emotional health. It can deplete a child's *qi*, *blood* and, in extreme cases, his *yin*. Qi deficiency might cause a temporary feeling of lowness. *Blood* and *yin* deficiency, however, mean that the *shen* is no longer properly 'housed' and this pathology is often involved in more long-term low feelings, as well as agitation and anxiety (see Chapter 12).

A child has a huge amount of *yang* and this means that he has a need to move and be active. However, his *yin* is insubstantial, which means that he needs to balance the need for movement with a lot of rest. It also means that if he does any kind of exercise that pushes him to dig deep into his reserves, it will deplete him. Growing, developing and building strong physical and emotional foundations should always be the top priority during childhood. Once a child has stopped growing, he then has basic building blocks from which he can springboard into refining his physical abilities through pushing himself a little harder.

How much is too much?

As Sun Simiao said, 'The way of nurturing life is to constantly strive for minor exertion but never become greatly fatigued and force what you cannot endure.'[2] As we have seen in other chapters, every child has a different constitution and therefore differing capacities for exercise. A strong, robust child may be able to tolerate playing his chosen sport three times a week and training on the days in between. However, for a child with a more delicate constitution, this amount of exercise would be depleting.

WHAT CAN WE DO TO HELP?

Children have extraordinarily different needs when it comes to exercise. The key is always to observe the individual child, rather than comparing them with another child. Take a look at Table 13.1, which will help guide you as to whether a particular child is getting insufficient exercise or is exercising excessively.

Table 13.1 Signs of over-exercise and insufficient exercise in a child

Signs of over-exercise	Signs of insufficient exercise
Moody, tearful or aggressive immediately after exercise	Tendency to be moody, grumpy or depressed when they have not exercised
Tired; lacking in bounce and energy; loses focus and becomes less productive for the rest of the day after exercise	Nevers stays still; always fidgeting or sluggish and lethargic which improves when they get moving
Chronic injuries	Wakes up feeling anxious or low and gets better with movement

A NOTE ABOUT TIREDNESS

Chinese medicine understands that, broadly speaking, there are two different causes of tiredness. The first is a deficiency condition, when the child's reserves of *qi*, *yin/yang* and/or *blood* are low. This type of tiredness is better for rest. The second cause is stagnation, when the flow of *qi* in the child's body is impaired. This type of tiredness is better for movement and exercise and does not improve with rest.

If a child often complains of feeling tired, it is helpful to determine which type of tiredness he has. A child with deficiency tiredness needs gentle exercise; a child with stagnation tiredness needs regular, more intense exercise and (crucially) feels less tired afterwards.

Of course, many children have a mixture of deficient and stagnant *qi*. As always, the right balance of rest and exercise needs to be found for each child.

Exercise to prevent and ease anxiety and depression

We will now look at the particular pathologies often involved in anxiety and/or depression, and discuss how exercise can either help or perpetuate them.

Qi stagnation

Check back to Chapter 7 to remind yourself about the nature of *qi* stagnation.

Qi stagnation is commonly found in a child who tends towards feeling low or depressed. His low feelings often comprise a sense of hopelessness, a feeling of 'can't be bothered' and a vision of the future that is bleak. He may feel tired much of the time but does not feel any better after sleep. He may resist getting out and doing something active but, when he does, he often feels better.

For the child with *qi* stagnation, exercise is not only important but absolutely crucial. Exercise helps to move *qi* in both the body and the mind. A child with *qi* stagnation might benefit from vigorous exercise several times a week. Jogging, dancing, playing football, swimming or any sport that involves lots of movement will help to keep his *qi* flowing. It might also benefit him to get out and move soon after getting up in the morning. Moving *qi* on waking can lift a child's mood for the rest of the day. It would therefore benefit this child to walk or cycle to school, for example.

Qi stagnation tends to become more pronounced premenstrually in girls. Exercise at this time of the month is a helpful way of managing symptoms of premenstrual tension.

Heat

Check back to Chapter 7 to remind yourself about the nature of *heat*.

An excess of *heat* in the body is often present in a child who is highly anxious and agitated. It may disturb sleep and make it hard for the child to relax and feel calm. Regular, gentle exercise that has a calming effect on the mind can help the *heat* to become dispersed. *Heat* is what is known in Chinese medicine as a secondary syndrome. It can arise as a result of a deficiency (usually of *yin*), in which case gentle exercise is appropriate. Or it can arise as a result of stagnation, in which case more intense exercise is appropriate.

Damp-phlegm

Check back to Chapter 7 to remind yourself about the nature of *damp-phlegm*.

Damp-phlegm is often present in a child who feels low and depressed. He may have a tendency to withdraw, want to sleep a lot and be rather unresponsive. *Damp-phlegm* is essentially a build-up of pathogenic fluids in the body, and movement is important to help to get the fluids circulating again. As with *heat*, gentle, rhythmic exercise is beneficial to resolve the *damp-phlegm*. However, underlying the build-up of *damp-phlegm* is often a lot of deficiency, which means that a child with *damp-phlegm* should avoid exercise that is too vigorous.

Blood deficiency

Check back to Chapter 7 to remind yourself about the nature of *blood* deficiency.

Blood deficiency is very common in children who are anxious and/or depressed, but it is especially common in adolescent girls. *Blood* deficiency often manifests with a mild, low feeling, a tendency towards feeling anxious, becoming easily tearful and having poor-quality sleep.

The onset of menstruation, lots of study and a poor diet all contribute towards *blood* deficiency. However, too much intense exercise is also an important contributory factor. At the most extreme end of the spectrum, this is seen in athletes who stop menstruating. However, it is common in many teenage girls who eat too little (see Chapter 15) and exercise too much in the quest for what they perceive to be the perfect body. During exercise, the *blood* is diverted to nourish the sinews and muscles and there is less available for the important role *blood* plays in helping to maintain mental/emotional equilibrium.

However, even a child who is *blood* deficient needs to exercise. The most suitable exercise in this case is gentle. Gentle yoga or simply walking involve enough movement to get the *qi* flowing, but do not strain the child's system.

It is also useful to talk to girls who are menstruating about differing needs for exercise at different times of the month. From the Chinese medicine perspective, girls should rest more and exercise less during and in the few days after menstruation. On the other hand, a little more exercise is useful in the premenstrual phase, when *qi* is prone to stagnate. Exercise in the premenstrual phase is especially helpful in girls who have a tendency to feel low or anxious at this time of their cycle.

Yin deficiency

Check back to Chapter 7 to remind yourself about the nature of *yin* deficiency.

Yin deficiency is often present in a child whose anxiety is on the extreme end of the spectrum. This child is likely to have a constant degree of anxiety and restlessness, to find it difficult to relax and to wake a lot during the night. Being *yin* deficient, ironically, can make a child feel that he is in overdrive and give an urge always to be active and on the go. This perpetuates the problem. Therefore, it is often difficult for a *yin*-deficient child to resist the urge to exercise vigorously, even though this will increase his level of depletion.

The best exercise for a child with *yin* deficiency is one that helps him to be grounded and that promotes stillness and calm. Traditional Chinese exercise such as *tai qi* and *qi gong* are particularly adept at this, but may not appeal to the *yin*-deficient child or, for that matter, to many children. In this case, the parent or practitioner needs to negotiate a reduction in the child's current levels of vigorous exercise, while at the same time discussing the benefits of other, more gentle forms of exercise.

The child who resists exercise

A lack of sufficient movement or exercise may become a cause of imbalance. A child who does not move his body enough will tend towards *qi* stagnation and *damp-phlegm*. As we saw in Chapter 12, these patterns are both common causes of low mood and depressive-type feelings. It is essential for a child or a teenager, both replete with *yang*, to have movement in his daily life. Yet it can also be difficult, especially as a child becomes older, to persuade him of this fact. In my paediatric clinic, every day I hear teenagers moan that their parents are always nagging them to get off their screens and get outside. And I hear parents moan that their teens are always inside on their phones and never get outside and move!

It is human nature to do something either because it is a necessity or because it is enjoyable. Understanding this is the key to finding creative ways for older children and teenagers to get up and moving. It is rarely effective to simply tell a teen that it will help him to feel better if he does more exercise.

WHAT CAN WE DO TO HELP?

- Teens and older children are very often motivated by the need to connect with friends, so finding a team sport with a friend or group of friends is a key motivating factor. It does not matter what the sport is, or whether or not he has a particular talent for it. If the fact that his friends do it gets him up and out, that is all that matters.

- For a child who finds competitive sport unappealing or even stressful, encouraging him to make an arrangement with a friend to go for a walk, cycle or meet in the skate park raises the chance of him doing it compared with doing it on his own.

- When safe and practical, withdraw offers of car rides so that it becomes a necessity for him to walk or cycle to school.

- Make it clear that incremental changes are great. If a teen thinks he has to become a long-distance runner to qualify as 'doing more exercise', that may put him off before he even starts.

- While lectures on the future benefits of exercise (helps prevent heart disease, osteoporosis, etc.) will likely fall on deaf ears, dropping into conversation the immediate benefits of exercise may help. Many children and teens do not know that exercise may help them to have more energy or sleep better, for example.

The child who exercises to excess

Qi stagnation, as we have seen, often leads to a low mood and depression. The reason that a child's mood often improves after exercise is that exercise moves *qi*, not only in the body but in the mind. Sometimes, more likely in the teenage years, a child finds himself becoming obsessive about exercise. It may have started out as something he did for pleasure, but becomes something he cannot do without, and feels the need to do more and more of in order to gain that 'feel-good' factor.

A child may also exercise obsessively as part of an eating disorder, such as anorexia. In these cases, exercise has switched from something that is health-giving to something that signals a deeper, underlying mental/emotional problem.

Qi stagnation may arise when a child feels chronically frustrated, angry or resentful. If exercise only gives him temporary relief from this feeling, or he has to do more and more of it to obtain the relief, then it is a sign that he needs help to get to the root of the problem.

WHAT CAN WE DO TO HELP?

- Support the child to connect with and acknowledge his intense feelings. Sometimes, creating opportunities for the right conversations can be enough. In some cases, getting help from a talking therapist is necessary.

- Explore what is causing the feelings. What is it about the child's life and his response to it that is evoking this level of intensity of emotion?

- Explore ways of reducing or eliminating the cause (when possible).

- Support the child to find other ways of expressing the feelings, e.g. through conversation or some creative outlet.

THE IMPORTANCE OF 'DOSAGE' WHEN IT COMES TO EXERCISE

Maggie began gymnastics classes when she was six and took to them like a duck to water. She loved the feeling she got when she elegantly moved her body in all sorts of wonderful ways. At age eight, Maggie was picked to train for a gymnastics club, and then at age ten she was chosen to train with the junior national team. This meant training five days a week, sometimes for up to four hours a day.

Maggie was brought to me for acupuncture treatment when she was fifteen. She had not yet begun menstruating but, more worryingly, over the last year she had begun to feel very low. She said she would become tearful for no apparent reason several times a day, cry herself to sleep at night, and had to dig deep to get out of bed in the mornings. When she was not at school or training, she would lie in bed feeling exhausted and depressed. She said she had no idea why, as she loved her life and gymnastics was everything to her.

Maggie had all the signs of extreme *blood* deficiency. When *blood* is deficient, the *shen* is not able to feel vital and alive, causing the low mood. Maggie's physical body had withstood the demands of her intense training well, but her spirit had suffered. With acupuncture treatment, a change in her diet and reduced training, Maggie started to feel a lot better. Her periods started too.

EXERCISE AS MEDICINE

Exercise is increasingly being prescribed by general practitioners, as part of the welcomed and growing trend of lifestyle medicine. As with any medicine, however, dosage is all-important.

In Chapter 16, we will talk about the wisdom of the traditional Chinese approach to eating (stopping eating when we are not yet quite full) being beneficial for health. The same rule applies to exercise. Stopping before reaching the point of exhaustion means that the child is not having to dig in to his reserves of *qi*. He is more likely to feel invigorated rather than tired for the rest of the day, and also more likely to keep up the exercise over a longer period of time.

A famous Jin dynasty scholar, Ge Hong, summed it up perfectly when he wrote, 'The body should always be exercised...yet even in exercise do not go to extremes.'[3]

WHAT CAN WE DO TO HELP?
Some general rules concerning what, where and how often

The best criteria for a child to choose which exercise will benefit him the most are:

- Which exercise lights his inner spark? If he does not enjoy it, he will not persist with it.

- How vigorous is the exercise relative to the strength of the child's constitution?

- Will the child's spirit be nurtured by doing a team sport that involves connection with other children? Or would he benefit more from exercise that is done alone where he can go inwards?

- Bearing in mind the constitution and nature of the child, would he benefit from training in his chosen sport five or six times a week? Or would that deplete him or make him feel pressured?

- Exercise in nature has many additional benefits. The Wood and Earth Elements, in particular, are nourished by being in a natural environment.

Seeing the wood for the trees

▶ Exercise is an important ingredient for good mental/emotional well-being.

▶ However, too much of the wrong type of exercise can be a contributory factor in poor mental/emotional well-being.

▶ The right amount and type of exercise for a particular child will depend on her patterns of imbalance. For example, a child with *qi* stagnation will require more vigorous exercise than one who is *qi* deficient.

Endnotes

1   Quoted in B. Flaws (2006) *A Handbook of TCM Paediatrics* (Boulder, CO: Blue Poppy Press), p. 7.

2   Sun Simiao, *Bei Ji Qian Jin Yao Fang* [Essential Prescriptions for Every Emergency Worth a Thousand in Gold], translated in S. Wilms (2010) 'Nurturing life in classical Chinese medicine: Sun Simiao on healing without drugs, transforming bodies and cultivating life', *Journal of Chinese Medicine* 93: 5–13, p. 10.

3   Ge Hong, *Inner Chapters of the Master Who Embraces Simplicity (Baopuzi yangsheng lun)*, in L. Kohn (2012) *A Source Book in Chinese Longevity* (St Petersburg, FL: Three Pines Press), p. 37.

Chapter 14

Breathing

The big picture

Breathing techniques have always been a key part of Chinese health practices. In the West, only recently have they become recognised as a way of improving health and, in particular, of managing anxiety.

The reason breathing can have such a powerful impact on a child's mental/emotional state is because it is a way of managing the flow of *qi* within the body. Anxiety and other intense feeling states can be understood, on one level, simply as disordered *qi*. Breathing has the power to bring *qi* back to a state of balance when it has been disrupted.

Breathing is not only essential to life but also plays a huge part in determining how a child grows, her vitality levels, her physical health and, most importantly, her mental/emotional health. Although it is something that a child does unconsciously, the Chinese understood that it is also something that we can control in order to improve the way we do it. We might think it strange that we should need to work on or improve such a fundamental bodily process. However, most of us do not grow up breathing in an optimal way.

When a child breathes well, it has the following benefits:

- It helps to regulate the *qi*.

- It helps to promote the free flow of *qi* in the body, which guards against *qi* stagnation.

- It helps to strengthen the Lungs and the Metal Element.

- It helps to calm the *shen*.

Each of these effects helps to relieve depression and ease anxiety. There is both a short- and a long-term benefit to breathing well. In the short term, breathing exercises can help a child who is experiencing acute anxiety, and sustained good breathing can have a lasting impact on a child's mental/emotional state.

What does 'good' breathing entail?
Breathe deep

'Good' breathing involves taking the movement of the breath deep down into the lower abdomen and lower back, as opposed to shallow breathing, when the movement does not extend beyond the chest. It is helpful for a child to rest a hand on her abdomen and imagine a balloon there that fills up with air as she breathes in.

Breathe slow

Slow breathing helps the breath to align with the metabolic needs of the body. It also has an especially calming effect on the mind. Aiming for a particular number of breaths per minute can be counterproductive, actually creating stress as the child feels she has to achieve a particular goal. It is more helpful to encourage a child to have times throughout the day when she focuses on her breathing and slows it down.

Breathe through the nose

In the Chinese tradition, it is considered more health-giving to inhale through the nose. This warms the air before it hits the lungs, which are susceptible to the effects of cold air. Warm air relaxes the *qi* and helps it to keep flowing smoothly, compared with cold air, which causes *qi* to contract. The exhale, therefore, is not as important and this can be done through either the nose or the mouth.

Nasal breathing has such a profoundly calming effect on a child's *shen* that it is worth persisting to train a child to breathe through her nose. Ironically, it is especially helpful for children who suffer from chronic nasal congestion and, unless the congestion is extreme, it is usually possible for a child with a blocked nose to breathe through her nose.

Breathing exercises

There are so many different breathing exercises suggested in books, on apps and in YouTube videos that it can become difficult for a parent or practitioner to know where to start supporting a child to breathe in a health-giving way. I have found the ones suggested below are easy for children to follow, but any exercise that encourages deep, slow nasal breathing will be helpful.

A word of caution, however. The aim is for a child's breathing to become naturally slower, deeper and nasal. The very idea of doing exercises to achieve this is somewhat contradictory to the ultimate aim of it occurring without needing to be forced. However, as with most skills in life, some time and effort usually needs to be put in. My suggestion would be for a child (with or without her parents, depending on age) to spend a few minutes twice a day practising breathing. An older child can be encouraged to focus on her breathing at other times too, such as when she is sitting in a lesson or in the car. Over time, slower, deeper and nasal breathing will gradually become the child's norm.

Breathing to help in the moment

These exercises can also be used in acute situations, such as before an exam or a social engagement. They can also be done if a child starts to feel herself becoming anxious or panicky at any point during the day or night. Focusing on the breath and slowing it down is one of the most useful strategies to get through a panic attack.

Breathing before bedtime

Another useful time to do these exercises is just before a child goes to bed, as they can help to calm the *shen* and promote a good night's sleep. Many parents have reported back to me that a couple of minutes spent focusing on the breath has become as much a part of their child's bedtime routine as cleaning their teeth or having a goodnight story.

Breathing in the long term

However, the goal is to encourage a child to have long-term, good breathing habits. Therefore, I urge parents to find a way of making these exercises a part of their child's daily routine over the long term.

Alternate nostril breathing

This exercise comes from the Indian yogic tradition. It reduces the level of sympathetic stress, which in Chinese medicine terms equates to the idea of calming the *shen*.

- Close the right nostril by placing the thumb over it.

- Inhale deeply and slowly through the left nostril.

- At the top of the breath, place the index finger over the left nostril, so that both nostrils are closed, and pause briefly.

- Lift the thumb off the right nostril.

- Exhale slowly through the right nostril.

- At the bottom of the breath, close both nostrils again and pause briefly.

- Repeat five to ten times.

Box breathing

This technique can be done by the child without anybody knowing she is doing it. It is also really simple even for young children to do on their own. It helps to bring a sense of calm and focus.

- Inhale through the nose to the count of 4.

- Hold the breath for a count of 4.

- Exhale to the count of 4.

- Pause to the count of 4.

- Repeat five to ten times.

Seeing the wood for the trees

▶ Good breathing practices do not necessarily come naturally, and it will benefit a child to be supported in developing a health-enhancing way of breathing.

▶ Breathing well helps to protect against and ease anxiety and depression, because it impacts the flow of *qi* in the body and the *shen*.

▶ The three most important aspects of breathing to focus on are: breathe deep, breathe slow and breathe through the nose.

• Chapter 15 •

The Art of Eating

The big picture

If we were to ask whether a child's diet alone directly causes anxiety or depression, the answer would usually have to be 'no'. Poor mental/emotional health usually arises when a combination of factors come together. However, it is true to say that diet can influence a child's mental/emotional health. This is particularly the case when the child is already struggling, and he is likely to be more sensitive to what he eats.

As we have repeatedly seen throughout this book, good mental/emotional health is inextricably linked with good physical health. It is impossible to separate the two, the mind and body being part of the same whole. Diet is a fundamental pillar that supports the growth and health of every part of a child. In this way, it is a protective factor against anxiety and depression.

The ultimate aim is to help a child develop a sense of what suits him, so that he chooses to eat what he can digest well and efficiently. As parents and practitioners, we sometimes need to put our own preconceptions about what the right and wrong foods and ways of eating are to one side. This chapter does not, therefore, propose a specific diet. It suggests a framework, within which parents and practitioners can create the right context to support a child to eat in a way that nourishes him.

The Chinese medicine view

Chinese medicine has always understood that diet is fundamental to health. The *qi* of the Stomach is said to be the source of life, and it supplies all the other organs in the body with *qi*. In fact, diet is considered a branch of medicine in its own right. A Chinese proverb states that 'He who takes medicine and neglects diet wastes the skills of the physician.' Anybody visiting an acupuncturist or Chinese medicine physician will probably be given suggestions for changes they may make to their diet that will support their return to health. The unique and wonderful power of Chinese dietary therapy is that it does not have blanket rules or a one-size-fits-all approach, but tailors its advice to suit the specific needs of the individual.

Diet is considered especially important for children because a child's digestive system is still developing. A little too much food, or a little of the wrong food, may be enough to throw things off balance. If this happens once in a while, it should not have any long-term consequences. Problems arise when a child eats too much of the wrong thing day after day. This can cause imbalances of *qi* that then have a direct and significant impact on a child's mental/emotional well-being.

The detail
How much to eat

When I was a child, my siblings and I were not allowed to leave the table until we had finished everything on our plate. This is an experience which will resonate with many readers. The norm in the West is to eat until we are full. The Chinese have long had a different idea (and one that modern science now supports) that is summed up in the Chinese saying 'When eating, stop when you are seven-tenths full.'

Babies and young children are particularly prone to the effects of eating too much. Chinese medicine describes one of the most commonly seen conditions in babies as 'food accumulation disorder'. It arises when the amount of milk or food ingested is too great for the digestive system to process. Food then lingers in either the stomach or intestines and begins to ferment. This creates *heat* in the body which then often rises up and affects the *shen* of the baby or young child. As a one-off, this is of little long-term consequence. If this pattern persists over a matter of years, it may lead to a child who has a chronic pattern of excess *heat* which, as we saw in Chapter 7, is commonly seen in children who are anxious.

It is easy to think that it would be impossible to overfeed a purely breastfed baby. However, Chinese medicine does not hold this view. The much-quoted 7th-century Sun Simiao wrote that 'Whenever you are breastfeeding a baby, you never want them to eat until they are too full. Overeating results in retching and vomiting... Nurse them on an empty breast, to make the [already ingested] milk disperse.'[1]

Even with breast milk, the baby's digestive system needs time to process one feed before he takes in another, in order to avoid 'food accumulation'.

However, it is not only babies and toddlers who suffer from the effects of eating too much. From the Chinese medicine perspective, digesting food consumes *qi*. This is *qi* that would otherwise be used to nourish a child's mind and brain. Another Chinese saying warned parents to be 'caring of the child, and sparing of its diet'. Simply put, eating too much consumes too high a proportion of a growing child's resources, and his mental/emotional health may be the part of him that suffers the consequences.

How much is too much?

This obviously begs the question of 'how much is too much?' Just as with everything else, each child needs a different amount of food. And each child has different dietary needs depending on his stage of life and the demands of his daily life. It is helpful to switch our focus from a particular quantity of milk or number of calories and instead look at the child to see if they are thriving on how much they are eating.

WHAT CAN WE DO TO HELP?

- A baby, even one who is breastfed, will usually benefit from a gap of at least two hours between the end of one feed and the start of the next.

- It is usual, and not a cause for concern, that a baby or child might have phases when he is more hungry and phases when he is less hungry. For example, babies often eat less when they are teething, which helps to make the process smoother.

- It is a wise strategy to serve small portions and allow a child to ask for more, compared with serving a bigger portion and expecting the child to finish everything on his plate.

When to eat

Eat more in the morning; less in the evening

While our parents may have been misguided in admonishing us for not finishing what was on our plates, they were spot on in telling us to 'breakfast like a king, lunch like a prince and dine like a pauper'. The *qi* of the Stomach and Spleen, which are responsible for a large part of the digestive process, is at its strongest between approximately 7 a.m. and 11 a.m., and at its weakest between the same hours in the evening. The human body mirrors the outside world, in that there is an abundance of *yang* at the start of the day and a maximum of *yin* in the evening and during the night. One ancient Chinese text explains: '*Yang qi* is swelling at noon and deficient at sunset; therefore more food should be taken for breakfast and less food for supper, and at night it is necessary to keep the stomach empty.'[2]

This means that a child needs and expects to get a good meal in the morning, and will be able more effectively to digest food at this time. A heavy meal in the evening will often be left partially digested, sit around in the digestive system overnight, interfere with sleep and mean the child is then not so hungry the next morning.

When a child reaches the teenage years, he may be less inclined to eat breakfast for various reasons. He may simply not get out of bed with enough time to eat, feeling his priority is sleep. Or he may find he is less hungry at this time of day than he used to be. This can, in itself, be a sign that his Earth Element (which governs digestion) has become depleted by having to process his increased food intake, too much of the wrong type of food and too much study. Yet if he can be supported to find a way to eat something at breakfast, it plays such a vital role in setting him up for the day. It will boost his mood and his brain power, and raise the chances of him eating in a more balanced fashion throughout the rest of the day.

WHAT CAN WE DO TO HELP?

- Encourage all children to have a substantial and nutritious breakfast.

- If a teenager is resisting eating anything in the morning, and all efforts to persuade him have failed, send him to school with something he can eat at his first opportunity during the morning.

- Having supper early in the evening (ideally three hours before bed-time) will increase the chances of a teenager eating in the morning, as well as helping sleep and protecting the *qi* of the digestive system.

Avoid snacking

The body needs long periods unoccupied with physical digestion in order for the mind to be able to tackle its thoughts and feelings. We have mentioned before that, according to the Chinese tradition, the separation of mind and body is an artificial one. This concept applies to digestion also. The process of digestion encompasses not only what the body does with food but what the mind and brain do with feelings and thoughts.

We have come to believe, as a society, that if a child does not eat something every couple of hours, he will faint or not cope in some way. Many children in the developed world do not know what it feels like to be hungry. However, if a child snacks throughout the day, there is less *qi* available for the mental and emotional aspects of the digestive process. This is not conducive to a calm and contented mood. The digestive system benefits from rhythm and routine, from meals at regular times and from avoiding snacking between mealtimes.

WHAT CAN WE DO TO HELP?

- Encourage a habit of eating properly at mealtimes.

- A child is less likely to eat well at mealtimes if he is not hungry because he has been snacking.

- Snacking can become a habit. Parents may need to support a child to break this habit, by modelling good eating habits themselves and perhaps not making snacking foods so easily available around the house.

- Snacking is rarely due to hunger, but commonly due to boredom, or a way of relieving difficult emotions. If a child can be taught to make friends with his feelings (as discussed in Chapter 8) it lessens his drive to snack.

How to eat

Eating should be pleasurable

Food is about more than nutrients. It is also a source of flavour and therefore pleasure. Taking time to eat, and doing so in a mindful way, can be a calming, mood-boosting experience. If a child grows up merely seeing food and eating as a means to an end, he is missing out on a potential source of satisfaction. We need to teach children to relish food.

When eating, just eat

As mentioned before, the Chinese consider digestion to be about a lot more than food. The *qi* a child uses to digest his food is the same *qi* he uses to digest the many experiences he has throughout the day. If a child is simultaneously eating and reading, studying or browsing on his phone, not only does he digest his food less well but he gets less pleasure from the experience of eating (see 'Eating should be pleasurable' above). When a child eats, his digestive *qi* needs to be in his intestines, not in his head.

The eating atmosphere

Just as digestion is about more than just food, mealtimes are about more than simply eating. They are an opportunity to connect, a time when a family can come together and process their individual experiences through conversation. Mealtimes can, potentially, be like a kind of coming back to the base and recharging, a *yin*-building experience after the *yang* activities of the day.

However, of course, we all know that mealtimes can also be a source of tension for a family, a time when the underlying dynamics rise to the surface and get played out. Battles over food are often not really about the food, but food has become the means through which wider issues are expressed.

A child's emotional state when he eats has an impact on how he digests his food. If a child is tense because of the family atmosphere, or any other reason, his Liver *qi* tends to stagnate. Liver *qi* must flow smoothly in order for the digestive process to work effectively. So conflict and tension at mealtimes hampers digestion. If digestion is impaired, this has a negative impact on a child's emotional state, as stagnant Liver *qi* is also commonly involved when a child is anxious and/or depressed.

As well as conflict, too many rules and expectations about what a child eats can mean that mealtimes are a time that he dreads. While of course a child needs to learn how to sit at mealtimes, eat sensibly and sometimes eat a little of what he does not relish, the many benefits of eating together as a family are wiped out when the child feels stressed or anxious about mealtimes.

Ideally, food should not really be the focus at mealtimes, but rather the focus should be on the communal aspect of eating together. Ironically, it is often when the focus on what and how much a child eats becomes too great that a child develops a less healthy relationship with eating.

WHAT CAN WE DO TO HELP?

- Involve children in the process of buying and cooking food from an early age.

- Give a child an opportunity to choose his favourite meal on a regular basis.

- Make some mealtimes an occasion rather than a rushed event.

- As parents, model putting away devices or other distractions at mealtimes, so that the focus is on the communal aspect.

Seeing the wood for the trees

▶ Getting into the habit of stopping eating before they are full can have a positive impact on a child's mental/emotional well-being.

▶ It will support a child's mental/emotional state to eat more in the morning and less in the evening, and to avoid eating within a couple of hours of going to bed.

▶ Constant snacking may have a negative impact on a child's emotional state.

▶ When eating is a pleasurable experience, it can support good mental/emotional health.

▶ If a child is, for example, on a device or doing homework while eating it will not only compromise their ability to digest their food but also lessen the chances of them relishing the experience of eating.

▶ Mealtimes are an opportunity for connection and for coming together as a family.

Endnotes

1   S. Wilms (trans.) (2013) *Venerating the Root: Part 1*. Sun Simiao's *Bei Ji Qian Jin Yao Fang*, Volume 5: Paediatrics (Corbett, OR: Happy Goat Productions), p. 81.

2   Cao Tingdon (1699–1785), *Common Sayings in Gerontology*, in L. Kohn (2008) *Chinese Healing Exercises: The Tradition of Daoyin* (Honolulu, HI: University of Hawaii Press).

Chapter 16

What to Eat

The big picture

Many books have been written entirely about what children should eat. Fashions come and fashions go about the best foods with which to wean a baby, whether or not children should eat red meat or soy, for example, or the optimal amount of green vegetables.

Undoubtedly, what a child eats is of importance and has consequences for his health. However, when what a child eats becomes more important than how much, when and how he eats, it is counterproductive.

From the Chinese medicine perspective, the old adage of 'we are what we eat' is not really true. We are what we make of what we eat. And what we make of what we eat depends on when we eat, how we feel when we are eating and how much we eat. It also depends on the condition of our digestive system which, in Chinese medicine, correlates to the Stomach and Spleen organs and the Earth Element.

On top of this, different children thrive on different diets. As with everything else we have discussed in the book, diet should be adapted according to a child's individual constitution. One child might tolerate a substantial amount of dairy in his diet, while it may make another child lethargic and sleepy. There is no universal, optimal diet, and part of the job of a parent or practitioner is to support a child in tuning in to his body and developing a sense of foods that are beneficial and those that are not.

Therefore, all the information in this chapter should be taken as guidelines rather than rules. They might help you to start homing in on some key food groups and the effect they may be having on a particular child. However, once again I urge you to take each child as an individual and focus on observing the effect their diet is having on them.

FOOD ENERGETICS

Whereas science tends to categorise foods according to the nutrients they contain, Chinese medicine understands food according to the effect it is likely to have on a person's *qi*. This is usually called the 'energetics' of food. For example, red meat is considered to have a slightly heating effect, and therefore too much of it might not suit a child who already has an excess of *yang*. On the other hand, red meat is also understood to nourish *blood*, and therefore would likely be beneficial for a child who is *blood* deficient.

Although certain foods have an inherent energetic quality, and a strong tendency to produce a particular effect on a child's *qi*, the focus should always be on observing how an individual child responds to a particular food. For example, too much sugar can mean one toddler becomes hyperactive, and another may become sleepy. The differing responses to the same food are due to the different natures of the two children's existing *qi*.

Some general guidelines
Variety

When it comes to diet, variety really is the spice of life. If there were just one principle to follow above all others, it would be to give a child the opportunity to eat as wide a range of largely healthy foods as possible. This principle of variety applies not simply to food types, but to taste. Of course, eating a wide range of fruit, for example, is more health-giving than eating only grapes. However, the aim is to eat some foods that are sweet, some that are bitter, some that are pungent and some that are sour. Foods of only one taste will create an imbalance of *qi*; foods of differing tastes will help to create harmony.

Lightly cooked foods

Cooked foods are much easier to digest than raw foods. Therefore, even though raw foods may contain more nutrients, the body is less able to assimilate them. This is especially true for a child, whose Stomach and Spleen needs to work doubly hard to break down uncooked food. However, overcooking saps foods of its *qi* and therefore its strengthening and building properties. Short cooking methods, such as lightly steaming and stir-frying, generally hit the middle ground that we are aiming for. The exceptions are roasting and slow-cooking stews and casseroles, which do not leach goodness out of the food.

Avoid cold foods and drinks

Chinese medicine stresses the importance of avoiding putting cold into the digestive system, which slows down the digestive process. There needs to be some digestive 'fire' in order for the body to effectively deal with food. We should try to encourage a child to say no to ice in his drinks, drinking or eating straight from the fridge and eating too much ice cream (except in hot weather or after a warm meal).

Specific food groups

The following section mentions just a few foods that, when they form a substantial part of a child's diet, may be a contributory factor to poor mental/emotional health.

Dairy

Dairy products (especially cows' milk products) are understood to clog up the *qi*, and have a tendency in many children to cause a build-up of *damp-phlegm* in the body. As we saw in Chapter 7, *damp-phlegm* increases the tendency of a child to become low and has a depressing effect on his spirit. It is as if the excess fluids literally put out the Fire of the child, meaning that it becomes difficult for him to feel any internal spark.

Fifteen-year-old Jason had begun to struggle with low mood over the last few months. It took three or four goes to wake him up and get him out of bed every morning. He walked to school in a complete daze and frequently fell asleep during classes. He said that everything felt like an effort and as if he was wading through treacle. He did not feel that anything in his life was fun any more. Jason used to play football but he had stopped that. It was on a Saturday morning and he said he'd prefer to be able to stay in bed. Evenings were his best time. They were the only time he actually felt awake and slightly enlivened.

Jason had always had a good diet at home. Since going to secondary school, he had more freedom in terms of what to eat. For his school lunch, he chose cheesy chips (deep-fried French fries covered in melted cheese) and a couple of slices of cheese pizza every single day. After school, he and his friends would go to the shop and buy waffles topped with chocolate sauce.

From a Chinese medicine perspective, Jason had too much *damp-phlegm* in his system. This was what was literally dampening down his mood and making him feel heavy, lethargic and sleepy. His teenage diet was now full of *damp-phlegm*-forming foods. While his friends seemed to be able to eat this without any obvious ill effects, Jason's constitution was different and he could not tolerate this diet.

Jason was resistant to changing what he ate and did not really believe there was a connection between that and his mood. However, over the month-long Christmas holidays, Jason reverted to his mum's healthy, home-cooked food. After the first couple of weeks, he began feeling more energetic, sleeping less and even going to kick a football around at the park with his friends again. When his mum pointed out to him that his change in diet was the most likely reason for the improvement in his mood, he reluctantly agreed there was probably a connection!

Sugar

For all but the most sensitive of children, a little sugar now and then will do little harm. Unfortunately, the diet of many children contains not just a little sugar, but significant quantities of it at every meal. Refined sugar is hidden in so many foods that it takes a concerted effort to avoid it.

For some children, sugar tends to create *heat*, and for others it tends to weaken the *qi* and lead to *damp-phlegm*. As we saw in Chapter 7, *heat* is commonly present in an anxious child and *damp-phlegm* is commonly present in a depressed child. However, beyond these energetic effects, eating too much sugar has bigger consequences. It means that a child's taste buds become habituated to excessively sweet foods, which in turns means he is less likely to enjoy foods of a more bitter or pungent flavour. Over time this can limit the variety in a child's diet.

Additives

I became aware of the strong impact additives can have on the sensitive system of a child when my eldest daughter was three years old. She was given a sweet that fizzed up in her mouth after lunch, and for the rest of the day she morphed from her generally cheery self to being angry, upset and inconsolable. I remember thinking at the time that some children eat these kinds of sweets frequently. This is an extreme example, but there is no doubt that, for some children, many commonly used food additives have a substantial and negative impact on their mental/emotional health.

Additives, which includes food colourings, preservatives and flavourings, tend to agitate the *qi* of a sensitive child, in particular the *qi* of the Liver. They may contribute to a child feeling irritable or hyperactive, or behaving aggressively.

WHAT CAN WE DO TO HELP?

- As always, the key is to observe. If a child's mood changes very suddenly, think back over the last half hour. There may be many triggers, but consider what he has eaten and note it down. You may start to see a pattern emerge.

Heavily processed foods

From a Chinese medicine perspective, heavily processed foods are empty calories. They have had the *qi* processed out of them. Unless they are full of additives (which they often are), they may not do much harm. However, they will not do any good either. They lack the ability to nourish, build and strengthen a child's body.

'Mono' or 'beige' diets

Some young children exist on a very narrow range of foods, often of the beige variety. Breakfast may be sugary cereal or white bread, lunch a white bread sandwich and supper white pasta or pizza. The child may eat a lot, but a lot of only one or two things. As we discussed earlier, too much food may overstretch the *qi* of the digestive system. Too much bland and processed food is even more detrimental, as it places a strain on the digestive *qi* but simultaneously does not nourish *qi* and *blood*.

Lack of *blood*-nourishing foods in menstruating girls

The lead-up to and when a girl starts menstruating is a time of enormous shift in the *qi* dynamics of the child. It is also commonly a time when mental/emotional problems arise. This is often because *blood* deficiency (see Chapter 2) sets in, as a result of monthly blood loss. This may often combine with other lifestyle factors that deplete *blood* such as excessive study, excessive exercise and poor diet. It is therefore crucial that during these years, a girl has a diet rich in *blood*-nourishing foods. These include:

- good-quality protein (either red meat, chicken, eggs or fish)

- green vegetables

- beetroot

- sweet potatoes

- lentils

- tofu

- molasses.

Blood-nourishing foods overlap with, but are not entirely the same as, foods that are rich in iron. As mentioned previously, Chinese medicine is not so focused on individual nutrients, but more on the energetic nature of food. Some foods are considered *blood* nourishing but may not, from the scientific point of view, be considered especially rich in iron.

Foods for patterns of imbalances often seen in anxiety and depression

If a child already has an imbalance, then it is a good idea to include, for a period of time, a greater quantity of foods with energetics that will help to address that particular imbalance. For example, if the child you have in mind is *blood* deficient, it will help her to have more *blood*-nourishing foods in her diet. If she has too much *damp-phlegm*, it will help her to avoid *damp-phlegm*-forming foods and include foods that help to ameliorate *damp-phlegm*.

On the other hand, in a healthy child, the most important thing is to support her to develop the art of eating, as outlined in the previous chapter, and to follow the more general guidelines outlined already in this chapter.

Qi stagnation

Foods to embrace: small amounts of citrus fruits (including the zest); pickled foods; buckwheat; rice; barley; carrots; herbs such as coriander, cumin, cardamom, fennel, basil and mint; vinegar; onions; garlic; small amounts of chicken and fish; pulses cooked with digestive herbs such as ginger and nutmeg.

Beneficial eating habits: avoid overeating, move after eating.

Foods to limit: deep-fried foods, oily foods, fatty meat, sugar, dairy food, chocolate, food additives (preservatives, colourings and flavourings).

Blood and *yin* deficiency

Foods to embrace: leafy green vegetables, beetroot, avocado, sesame seeds, pumpkin seeds, dates, apricots, good-quality organic animal products, almonds, lentils.

Beneficial eating habits: regular meals, eat slowly, when eating focus on eating, avoid eating late in the evening.

Foods to limit: coffee, alcohol, hot and spicy foods, low-protein diets.

Damp-phlegm

Foods to embrace: barley; rye; corn; buckwheat; rice; fresh ginger; spices such as pepper, cardamom, nutmegs and cloves; garlic; celery; pumpkin; apples; citrus zest.

Beneficial eating habits: avoid overeating, don't drink at mealtimes, move after eating.

Foods to limit: dairy, oily or fatty foods, sugar, peanuts and peanut products, yeasted products, orange juice, bananas.

Heat

Foods to embrace: watermelon, cucumber, apples and pears, lettuce, oats, yoghurt.

Beneficial eating habits: eat a small amount in the evening, ensure mealtimes are calm.

Foods to limit: spices, red meat, coffee, onions and garlic, alcohol, recreational drugs.

WHAT CAN WE DO TO HELP?

- Look back to Chapter 7 to remind yourself of which particular pattern of imbalance you think predominates in the child you have in mind.

- Look at the child's diet over a week and make a list of foods that it might benefit them to reduce, and foods that it might benefit them to eat more of.

- Over time, gradually tweak the child's diet (or support the parent to do the same) so that it better supports her mental/emotional health.

- With the exception of strong trigger foods, it is what she eats overall during weeks and months, rather than the odd lapse, that will make the most difference.

Diets

Dieting often crops up in the teenage years, especially, though not solely, in girls. As well as usually being ineffective as a way of achieving long-term weight loss, repeated and/or fad dieting is commonly a symptom of underlying unhappiness.

There is often a misguided underlying assumption that 'If I were thinner, I would be happy.' Dieting often makes the situation worse. It can create a roller coaster of emotion; the temporary high of seeing the pounds drop off, and the ensuing low when they pile back on. Dieting is also like the curse of Sisyphus, as when the girl reaches her desired weight she finds that longed-for contentment is still elusive.

Diets may also be a way of disconnecting from an uncomfortable emotion. As we saw in Chapter 8, trying to avoid a feeling does not mean that it goes away but, on the contrary, makes an equitable mental/emotional state more difficult to achieve.

On top of this, diets that exclude what Chinese medicine terms *blood*-nourishing foods lead to or exacerbate *blood* deficiency. A common symptom of *blood* deficiency is anxiety.

Eating and feeling

Although no parent intends this, many children are brought up to use food as a way of managing emotions. A nice, sugary treat is offered to a child as a way of consoling him when he is hurt or upset. Food may be given to a child as a reward for behaving well or performing well at school. It may even be given as a substitute for love and affection, when the parents are not at ease with displaying these emotions. Sugary foods are denied to a child because he has been naughty. In some children this may lead to unhelpful eating patterns.

I have seen many teenagers in my clinic who use food to escape feelings that are difficult, either by denying themselves food or by comfort eating. As we saw in Chapter 8, if a child tries to escape a feeling, the feeling then disturbs the movements of *qi* and the *shen*. The wonderful children's book *We're Going on a Bear Hunt* by Michael Rosen could have been referring to emotions when it says, 'We can't go over it. We can't go under it. Oh no! We've got to go through it!'[1]

Eating disorders

An in-depth discussion of eating disorders is beyond the scope of this book. However, they do need mentioning, because an eating disorder often arises out of an underlying state of anxiety and/or depression. At the root is a feeling or feelings that have been heavily suppressed or from which a child has disconnected. One of these feelings may be anxiety. Or anxiety may come in the place of another feeling that the child has suppressed. When the feelings become too much to bear, the child may then begin to control his eating (as in the case of anorexia) or compulsively eat, both being attempts to numb the anxiety and/or depression.

When a child has treatment that tries to prevent the unhealthy eating habits (e.g. in the case of anorexia, he is forced to eat a certain number of calories a day), although he may resume a healthier weight, what is often left behind are the intense feelings that led to the disordered eating in the first place. Unless the child has help to address these underlying feelings and states, although his eating habits may be considered healthy, he cannot be considered to be truly cured.

WHAT CAN WE DO TO HELP?

- The work of separating eating and emotion will ideally start from early childhood, by avoiding rewarding or punishing a child with food.

- In an older child, the best way to break this relationship between eating and feeling is to help a child make friends with her emotions, as outlined in Chapter 8.

Seeing the wood for the trees

▶ Chinese medicine is concerned predominantly with the effect a particular food has on a child's *qi*, rather than what nutrients it contains.

▶ Every child will need a different diet in order to thrive mentally/ emotionally, depending on their patterns of imbalance.

▶ Having said that, all children will benefit from having a varied diet, consisting largely of lightly cooked foods, and avoiding too many cold food and drinks.

▶ The food groups that most commonly negatively impact on a child's mental/emotional health are:

  – dairy foods

  – sugar

  – additives

  – heavily processed foods.

Endnote

1   M. Rosen and H. Oxenbury (1993) *We're Going on a Bear Hunt* (London: Walker Books), p. 2.

Chapter 17

Sleep

The big picture

Li Liweng (1611–1679) wrote that 'The secret of good health lies in a good and restful sleep… Is not sleep the infallible miracle drug, not just a cure for one illness but for a hundred, a cure that saves a thousand lives.'[1] Sleeping well is essential for good mental/emotional health. Sleeping badly is both a cause and a symptom of poor mental/emotional health. While this may appear to be a chicken-and-egg situation, from the Chinese medicine perspective, thinking of it as a straightforward cause and effect is to oversimplify. Poor sleep and poor mental/emotional health often co-exist and perpetuate each other, and which one came first is not really a question that it is usually possible or helpful to answer.

Good sleep is essential to maintain mental/emotional well-being, and disturbed sleep patterns (either an inability to sleep or a desire for excessive sleep) are common symptoms of anxiety and depression.

How much sleep does a child need?

Every baby and child is unique, and some have sleep needs that are different from others of a similar age. However, Table 17.1 shows the widely accepted guidelines for sleep requirements at different ages. If a child is getting a wildly different number of hours of sleep from the average at their age, it may indicate or contribute to a mental/emotional imbalance.

Table 17.1 Hours of sleep needed at different ages

Age	Hours of sleep needed per 24 hours	Daytime sleep (hours)	Night-time sleep (hours)
Newborns (0–3 months)	14–17		
6 months	14	3	11
1 year	13.5	2.5	11
2 years	13	1.5	11.5
3 years	11.5–12.75	0–0.75	11.5–12
4–9 years	11–12.5		11–12.5
10–16 years	9–12		9–12

Information taken from the Children's Sleep Clinic at http://millpondsleepclinic.com, January 2021.

The Chinese medicine view

Sleep has its basis in *yin*; daytime activity has its basis in *yang*. As we saw in Chapter 1, at the heart of Chinese medicine is the interplay between *yin* and *yang*. To remain in harmony with the cycles of *yin* and *yang*, a child manifests his *yang* through being active during the day. As night-time draws near, he connects with his *yin*, becoming peaceful, slowing down his mind and eventually falling asleep. It is while a child is in this deep, *yin* state that his mind and body are nourished and restored.

The *shen* is said to 'govern' sleep. If the *shen* is disturbed, sleep will not be good. There are several pathologies that may disturb the *shen*:

- *blood* deficiency

- *yin* deficiency

- *heat*.

We discussed these pathologies in Chapter 7. You might want to check back to that chapter now to refresh your memory.

Causes of poor sleep

An overloaded digestive system

In Chinese medicine, there is a strong link between sleep and the digestive system. The 17th-century doctor Zhang Jiebin wrote that 'When the stomach loses its harmony, one's sleep is not peaceful.'[2]

This correlation between sleep and digestion is particularly impactful in babies and young children, although it remains important throughout life. A parent may feel instinctively that having a good feed or meal in the evening means that their baby will sleep better, but this is not necessarily the case. A baby has a delicate digestive system and it is a mammoth task to digest all the milk and/or food he needs in order to grow. In Chapter 15, we discussed a pattern called food accumulation disorder, which arises from excessive food intake and which is a common cause of poor sleep in this age group.

Of course, poor sleep in the first year or two of life is exceedingly common and not necessarily a precursor to poor mental/emotional health as a child. On the other hand, a baby or toddler sleeping poorly often results in the parents becoming exhausted. This creates strain in the family which will, in turn, negatively impact the child.

The digestive system is more robust in older children and less easily affected by what the child eats. Having said that, an older child who has a sensitive digestion, or one who is not sleeping well for other reasons, usually benefits from several easy-to-implement changes to his diet and eating habits.

WHAT CAN WE DO TO HELP?

- Allow a minimum of two hours between the end of the evening meal and bedtime.

- Avoid sugary foods in the evening.

- Avoid spicy foods in the evening.

- Ensure that the eating environment is calm during the evening meal.

- Create opportunities for the child to do some gentle movement after the evening meal.

Rumination and worry

Disturbed sleep is often a continuation of worry, restlessness or anxiety during the day. Therefore, of overarching importance in the search for good sleep is the idea of stilling the mind, and therefore calming the *shen*. One ancient Chinese text says, 'Before going to sleep, first the mind must become calm.'[3]

The tendency to restlessly revisit thoughts and feelings, and to worry, 'knot' the *qi* and mean the mind and spirit of the child cannot sink down into a place of stillness and calm. This tendency often increases during adolescence, alongside greater pressures at school and added social pressures.

● WHAT CAN WE DO TO HELP?

- Give a child the opportunity to talk through her worries before she goes to bed. Alternatively, create a worry box, into which a child can put her worries before she goes to sleep. If she is old enough, she can write them down and put them in the box, or otherwise she can put beads or other small objects that represent her worries in the box.

- Remember that sleep is often a reflection of daytime life. Is there something in the child's life that is affecting her ability to sleep? If so, what can be done to modify or eliminate it?

Eleven-year-old Kacey had been taking a long time to get off to sleep for the last two or three months. She got into bed at a sensible time, but tossed and turned for hours before she was eventually able to drop off. She said that during these hours, her mind was whirring around and around, busy with lots of thoughts. She was also feeling increasingly anxious during the day.

Kacey was trying out for a scholarship for her next school. She was having additional tutoring sessions, and doing extra homework in preparation for the exam. It became obvious during our discussion that this was feeling like an enormous strain for Kacey. We talked this through with Kacey's parents. Everybody agreed that the strain the scholarship was placing on Kacey and the negative impact it was having on her sleep were simply not worth it. Thankfully, Kacey's parents realised that good mental/emotional health is far more precious than getting a scholarship.

Within a couple of weeks of pulling out of the scholarship, Kacey's sleep improved and her anxiety levels dropped.

Intense emotions

A key medical text explains that 'When the emotions have something they lean towards, then one lies down to sleep and cannot find rest.'[4] Intense emotions disturb and agitate the *shen*, leading to poor sleep. This is the case either when the emotions are expressed intensely or when they are repressed. The idea of emotions being a disruptive factor for a child's mental/emotional health was discussed in Chapter 8. We know as adults that going to sleep on an argument, or after watching a particularly adrenalising television programme late in the evening, can disturb our sleep. A child is even more susceptible to strong emotions disturbing her sleep.

WHAT CAN WE DO TO HELP?

- Be mindful of the emotional environment in the household in the evening. When parents and children are tired at the end of a long day, it is easy for tempers to fray and strong emotions to erupt. The more a parent is trying to rush a child's bedtime, the more likely it is for the child to resist going to bed. Parents reframing bedtime from being a tiresome chore to being an opportunity to connect with their child is sometimes enough in itself to transform a child's sleep patterns.

- Strong emotions are qualitatively *yang* in nature. The best way to temper *yang* is to respond to it in a *yin* manner. There is power in a *yin* approach, being as flexible and receptive as possible rather than being reactive to an overtired child or a stroppy teenager.

- If a teen is not sleeping because of intense emotions which are repressed, this requires a more long-term approach and possibly help from a professional such as an acupuncturist or therapist.

Screen time

We discussed screen time in Chapter 12. Apart from the fact that the blue light emitted from many devices delays the release of melatonin (a sleep-inducing hormone), we saw that many screen-time activities agitate the *shen*. This is particularly the case with time spent on social media.

The online social life of many teenagers comes alive in the evening, and a child often fears missing out. When an older child or teen is allowed to keep devices in his bedroom, his online world is often the first thing he thinks about in the morning and the last thing he thinks about before going to sleep. This does not allow for a gradual descent into a more *yin* state in the evening, or a gradual easing into daytime mode.

WHAT CAN WE DO TO HELP?

- Leaving a minimum of an hour between any prolonged bout of screen time and bedtime is a good aim.

- Screens should be kept out of the bedroom at night-time. If there is one screen-time rule that should not be compromised, this is it. And it should apply to everyone in the household (parents and children alike)!

Parents tell me time and time again that they have more battles over screens than anything else, and particularly about getting teens off their screens in the evening.

In an ideal world, the parent and teen will work together to come up with a plan, so the teen does not feel it has been forced upon them. This probably takes compromise on both sides. The aim is for the teen not to feel enraged about the limitations of her screen time in the evening but that the limitations are sufficient to promote good sleep, and are therefore understood as being beneficial for that reason.

Studying late in the evening

Studying encourages too much of the child's *qi* into her head and has a 'knotting' effect. This prevents the *shen* from being peaceful and jeopardises the chance of good sleep. A child who has studied right up until she tries to sleep may find that her thoughts are trapped in a circle and go around and around in her head, preventing her from dropping off.

WHAT CAN WE DO TO HELP?

- Leave some time between the end of studying and bedtime. Some gentle movement, such as walking, stretching or yoga, will encourage the *qi* to 'unknot' and come back down into the child's body.

Not enough exercise during the day

If a child does not move her body, and therefore her *qi*, during the day, it may lead to restlessness at night. Depending on the constitution of the child, her need for exercise will vary. Insufficient exercise leads to stagnant *qi*, which prevents the child's body from relaxing and being able to settle into sleep. An older child or teenager needs to be supported to adapt her daily schedule to incorporate an appropriate amount of exercise and movement to match her constitution.

WHAT CAN WE DO TO HELP?

- Encourage walking or cycling to school when possible.

- For children with high exercise needs, prioritise activities that allow for this.

- Create opportunities for a child to exercise in the morning, when *qi* is at its strongest. If the school schedule prevents this, then as soon after school as possible is the next best time.

- Avoid exercising too late in the evening, which can overstimulate and work against getting a good night's sleep.

Difficulty sleeping at different times of the night

Chinese medicine relates poor sleep at different times of night to specific Elements, as follows:

- Difficulty getting off to sleep in the evening tends to be related to the Fire Element.

- Waking up in the middle of the night and being wide awake (especially around 1–3 a.m.) tends to be related to the Wood Element.

- Waking up too early in the morning tends to be related to the Water Element.

Difficulty getting off to sleep

The evening and first part of the night is governed by the Fire Element. This gives us some clues as to what might be making it difficult for a child to drop off to sleep. First, the Fire Element needs connection and intimacy in order to remain balanced. A difficulty falling asleep may be a difficulty separating. For a Fire child, this impending separation may agitate him, either consciously or unconsciously. Feeling agitated makes sleep more difficult and staying awake means he can put off the separation he fears.

So, if a child struggles getting off to sleep and comes up with lots of reasons to keep coming downstairs or get his parents to keep coming upstairs, it is likely a Fire issue that is the problem. In particular, it tends to be *blood* and/ or *yin* deficiency affecting this Element.

WHAT CAN WE DO TO HELP?

To help a child get off to sleep, as well as the tips given earlier in this chapter, also:

- Ensure that the child has had good-quality interaction and connection with parents and other family members in the evening so that his 'intimacy bucket' will be fuller at bedtime, making it easier for him to separate.

- Avoid interaction that agitates or excites the child before bedtime. Fill the last few hours of the day with calm, communal and connected activities, whenever possible.

Waking in the middle of the night

The middle of the night, more specifically approximately between the hours of 1 a.m. and 3 a.m., is governed by the Wood Element, especially the Liver. So a child who consistently wakes up and stays awake during this time may have an imbalance in this Element. Nightmares, night terrors, excessive dreaming, sleep talking and sleep walking can all also be signs of trouble in the Wood Element.

When a child cannot sleep, a useful question to ask is what is going on in his head while he stays awake. If a child says he lies awake in the middle of the night thinking about everything he has to do the next day or making plans, that is another clue that the Wood Element is involved. As we saw in Chapter 4, the emotion connected with the Wood Element is anger. So, if a child says he lies awake in the middle of the night feeling furious about his parents' decision to increase his chores, or dwelling on a row he had with his sister, it is most likely a Wood imbalance that is keeping him awake.

WHAT CAN WE DO TO HELP?
To help a child to sleep through the night:

- Question whether an older child is feeling overloaded by his to-do list.

- Does the child have feelings of anger/frustration/resentment that he is not able to express for some reason? What would help him to discharge these feelings in an acceptable way during the day?

- Ensure the child's diet does not contain additives or an excess of sugar, both of which can agitate the Wood Element (see Chapter 16).

Waking early the morning
The hours of approximately 3 a.m.–7 a.m. are governed by the Water Element. If a child is prone to waking early, and is unable to get back to sleep, it may be because the *yin* of the Water Element is not strong. He may wake up needing to go to the loo but cannot get back to sleep again afterwards. He may also be prone to bed-wetting. He may feel exhausted, and that he has not had enough sleep, but simultaneously 'buzzy' and raring to go. Counterintuitively, if he missed his usual bedtime the evening before, or was 'wired but tired' when he went to bed, he is more likely to wake up earlier the next day. Feelings of anxiety or insecurity will also make him more prone to waking early. For example, if his parents were out and he was put to bed by someone he does not feel completely safe and familiar with, it can trigger an early waking.

WHAT CAN WE DO TO HELP?
To help a child to sleep later in the morning:

- What happens in the evening influences what happens in the morning, so keeping bedtime as calm as possible increases the chances of a child sleeping later in the morning.

- Do everything possible to make the child feel as secure as possible at bedtime.

- The more tired the child is when he goes to sleep, the more he is likely to wake early, so making sure bedtime is not delayed is helpful.

- Making sure the room is dark can encourage a child to sleep later in the morning.

A word about teenagers and sleep

The sleep patterns of teenagers are notorious for changing. Many teenagers struggle to get off to sleep at what their parents consider an acceptable time. Many also struggle to get up in the morning at what their parents consider an acceptable time! The explanation usually given for this is that the sleep-inducing hormone melatonin is released in the brain of teenagers later in the evening than it is for children and adults. Similarly, the hormone cortisol, which helps us to wake up, is released in the brain of a teenager later in the morning than in adults or children.

However, some neuroscientists now believe that these hormonal changes do not make as big a difference to sleep patterns as we once thought and that the changes are more brought about by the social context, such as the draw towards socialising on technology in the evening and the increase in worry.

Chinese medicine has its own explanation for these changes in the sleep patterns of teenagers. The first is that adolescence involves a surge in *yang*, which creates more *heat*, restlessness and wakefulness in the mind and body. The second is that the Fire Element (which, as we saw in Chapter 4, craves connection and intimacy) is at its height between the hours of 7 p.m. and 11 p.m. Regardless of their constitutional type, teenagers have an immensely strong biological drive to connect with their peers, and the need to do this will be at its strongest during these hours in the evening. The third is that the Earth Element is under strain during adolescence because it is responsible for processing the huge amounts of food teenagers consume to support their growth spurt. The Earth Element helps to send clear *yang* to the head to promote wakefulness and clear thinking. The time of the Earth Element is

7 a.m.–11 a.m., which is exactly the time teenagers often feel at their most sleepy and are most drawn to pulling the duvet over their heads and going back to sleep.

However, all is not lost. Following the suggestions made throughout this chapter can mean that a teen gets an extra hour or two's sleep at night, which can make the difference between her thriving rather than simply surviving.

Seeing the wood for the trees

▸ Good sleep relies on the *shen* being peaceful and calm.

▸ Poor sleep is both a cause and a symptom of anxiety or poor mental/ emotional well-being.

▸ Eating too much, or the 'wrong' foods, too close to bedtime can disturb sleep.

▸ Poor sleep can be a manifestation of separation anxiety.

▸ Worry and studying close to bedtime can 'knot' a child's *qi* and interfere with sleep.

▸ Intense emotions, either expressed or repressed, disturb the *shen* and negatively impact sleep.

▸ In older children and teens, screen time in the evening and a lack of exercise in the day may both prevent sound sleep.

Endnotes

1   *The Arts of Sleeping, Walking, Sitting and Standing*, in Lin Yutang (1961) *The Importance of Understanding* (London: Heinemann), p. 259.

2   P. Unschuld and H. Tessenow (2011) *Huang Di Nei Jing Su Wen: An Annotated Translation of Huang Di's Inner Classic – Basic Questions*, 2 volumes (Oakland, CA: University of California Press), p. 500.

3   *Secret of Sleep*, quoted in Liren Yuan and Xiaoming Liu (1992) 'Traditional Chinese methods of health preservation', *Journal of Chinese Medicine* 41: 32–37, p. 32.

4   *Jia Yi Jing*, Huang Fumi, in P. Unschuld and H. Tessenow (2011) *Huang Di Nei Jing Su Wen: An Annotated Translation of Huang Di's Inner Classic – Basic Questions*, 2 volumes (Oakland, CA: University of California Press).

Chapter 18

What Else Can We Do to Help?

Having read Part 2, and seen that good mental/emotional health arises out of the fabric of a child's life, you may be wondering where to start and what to do with the information you have just read. In this final chapter, I will outline some general principles which, I hope, will help you to help the children with whom you are concerned.

The art of the heart

It is a tenet of both Confucianism and Daoism that each person has in her life a 'contract with heaven'. This is a translation of the Chinese word *ming*. Our *ming* consists of a certain path through life, one in which we live according to our true nature and thus achieve our potential. If a person is connected to her *ming*, then she will feel that her life has meaning and purpose.

You might be thinking: what has this got to do with children? We cannot possibly expect a child to know what her true purpose in life is. Yet the ability as an adult to know one's *ming* largely stems from the circumstances of our childhood.

As parents, carers, practitioners or educators, we know that our primary role in a child's life is to support her to become a well-functioning, independent, contented adult. Yet we sometimes believe that, in order to do that, we need to focus on her school grades, her sporting prowess, her ability to keep her room tidy or to remember everything she has to take to school in the morning. Of course, these things do matter and do require attention. However, they are all of relatively minor importance compared with the task of 'obtaining oneself' (*ze di*) in order to be able to achieve one's *ming*.

How do we do this? In order to help a child achieve her *ming* in her adult life, the most important thing we can do is to recognise, accept and support her to live according to her true nature as a child. The more we are attached to our own hopes and expectations for a child, the more it obscures our view of a child's true nature.

The art of the heart is the idea of making the heart the centre of everything a child does. If something lights her spark on a consistent basis, it probably means that it is in accordance with her true nature. Of course, at times children have to do things they would rather not, and they have to get through boring times. However, it is essential that there is something that feeds their heart as a counterbalance.

If there is a common thread in the children I see who are struggling with their mental/emotional health, it is this. Their heart, their *shen*, their spirit is not being looked after. They may be living a life which looks from the outside to be wonderful. Yet it is not wonderful *for them*. Sometimes the smallest change – a little more time with a parent, a small easing of the daily schedule, a friend or teacher who they feel sees into their soul, a new activity that feels just right – is the magic that is needed in order for them to thrive.

Connection comes above all else

On his death bed, the great physician Sun Simiao wrote that people have illness 'because they do not have love in their lives and are not cherished'.[1] The number-one way to look after the *shen* of a child is to have connection and intimacy with her. However challenging a child may find it, however much a teenager may appear that she does not want or need it, being connected to other human beings is essential for a child's mental/emotional well-being. Of course, children of different Element types need varying types and degrees of connection. How we go about creating connection should be guided by this.

Creating connection is not a one-off event. It is something that needs continual work. As parents and practitioners, creating connection with the children for whom we care involves holding up a mirror to ourselves and sometimes facing some harsh truths about how we might be inadvertently sabotaging the quality of our connection. It involves the ability to be self-reflective, to be flexible and adaptable and to be adept at managing our own emotions in relation to the children for whom we care.

Being connected with a child does not mean always having complete harmony with her. Long-term relationships inevitably involve times of discord. However, it does mean a willingness to hold a child in our minds, to have a profound respect for her unique nature and a commitment to keep striving for connection even when it would be easier to disconnect. This in turn can enhance the quality of our connection and build trust between ourselves and a child, even when there may be periods of disharmony.

Connection is important for another reason too. A parent or practitioner will have much greater influence on a child when they have rapport. Trying to persuade a child to go to bed earlier or eat more vegetables will generally not be successful unless the child feels a relatively strong connection with the person doing the persuading. Confucius wrote that, 'If man asks for something without having first established relations, it will not be given to him.' My advice, therefore, would be to spend as much time as it takes working on connection before implementing any other changes you believe will be necessary.

The orchestra principle

I have had teenagers in my clinic say things like 'I don't do any exercise but that's OK because I eat well,' or 'I eat loads of junk food but I compensate for that by doing lots of exercise.' Unfortunately, life does not work like that. All the aspects of life we talked about in Chapter 8 through to Chapter 17 can be compared to instruments in an orchestra. If one is really out of sync with the others, it lets the whole side down. It is no good having a string section who excel if the woodwind section is hopeless. In order to build and maintain strong mental/emotional health, we need to support children to be mindful of all aspects of their lives. It is certainly not the case that everything has to be perfect, but everything does need to be good enough.

Coping with hard times

When life is relatively unstressful and going along quite smoothly, there is generally room for flexibility in how a child lives her life. A healthy child will probably be able to cope with some late nights during the summer holidays without there being any ill effects. Frequent late nights during term time and in the winter (when the child is expending more *qi* to get through the day and there is less available due to shorter daylight hours and a lack of sun) may be another matter.

It is much harder to make positive changes to how we live during stressful times. Therefore, the goal must be to instil good habits in the easy times that will then be naturally continued during harder times. When a child is doing important exams, changing schools, recovering from an illness or dealing with turbulence in her friendship group, there will be less slack in terms of how much pressure her system can cope with. Building a bank of good habits in easier times can pay off to support a child through tougher times.

Working together

Instilling healthy living in a child is not easy. When a parent is tired and at their wits' end, it is all too tempting to take short cuts. It is also extremely difficult to stick to something you believe is right for your child when every other child in the class seems to be doing something different. The outcome is likely to be far better if children are involved in decisions, rather than having decisions imposed upon them. It may lead to feelings of constraint and consequent anger, negatively impacting the Wood Element, when a child is told to do something 'just because' or if she feels constantly powerless.

A child will usually respond better if she sees that there is good reasoning behind something she is being asked to do or not do. Parents whose children live exemplary lives, but do so because they have been ruled with a rod of iron, are highly likely at some point to rebel or to suffer from mental/emotional difficulties because they have repressed so much emotion.

We want a child to make good choices not because she will suffer her parents' wrath if she doesn't, but because she believes it is in her best interests to do so. The aim is not to create highly compliant and obedient children but to nurture our children's ability to be self-aware and make sensible choices for themselves. Having said that, none of us learns what 'sensible' choices are without having made many mistakes along the way. Particularly in the teenage years, the most efficient way for a child to find out what helps him to thrive rather than hinders him is through experience. One of the many challenging aspects of parenting is to be able to stand back and allow the child to learn through doing.

Making decisions in the heat of the moment

It is all well and good to read this book, and think you have all the answers you need and know what to do. You then find yourself in the middle of a difficult moment with a child, full of emotion, berating yourself about how you handled it and then, afterwards, not having a clue how to move forward. For example, your child is upset and anxious as a result of what other children said to her in a heated online exchange that took place at midnight when you thought she was fast asleep. You have had so many discussions where she has told you she is going to come off social media, leave her phone downstairs and concentrate on her close friendships as she knows the online stuff heightens her anxiety. You feel despairing!

This is where the Daoist concept of *wu wei* becomes invaluable. This is a concept that is relatively easy to describe but takes practice and commitment to actually live. But it is never too late to start cultivating it. *Wu wei* is often translated as 'non-action'. However, what it actually means is to act in accordance with the nature of a particular time. It refers to action that is driven by the needs of the situation as opposed to the person's needs or desires.

To go back to our teenager and her phone, a parent may understandably feel they want to have a rant at their child about how she never seems to learn, and does she not want to help herself, etc., etc. However, that would be acting according to the parent's own need to discharge their frustration and upset which, while understandable, is most likely not helpful. Ironically, it is also likely to lessen the chances of the child 'learning her lesson' because in that moment, for the child, the whole event has become about her parent 'not getting it' and being cross or disapproving of her.

What does this situation really require? Most probably, the child needs her parent alongside her, in a calm state, as she deals with her upset and her probable frustration for getting herself into this situation again. Most probably, she needs to feel connected to her parent in order for her anxiety to be soothed. There may be a time later on when a discussion might prove useful, but the heat of the moment is rarely the right time for that.

I am not suggesting that we all need to parent as a Daoist sage would have done. That would inevitably set us all up for failure. However, when we hit up against these snags as we try to instil good habits in our children, employing the concept of *wu wei* can create an opportunity for a breakthrough.

Remaining endlessly curious

There will inevitably be times, as a practitioner or a parent, where you feel you just do not understand what is going on with a child. You can see that she is not thriving, but you are stuck as to why that might be. If you find yourself in this situation, I urge you to put aside any assumptions you may have about the child or their situation and develop your curiosity. For example, one parent told me she was absolutely sure her son was withdrawn and low because for the first time in his life he was no longer top of the class in all his subjects. In fact, it turned out he was not in the least bit bothered about that. What had really affected his mood was the fact that he felt he was so tall and thin, and he wanted to be muscly and athletic-looking. As a result of his parents making wrong assumptions as to the cause of his mood, any conversations they had with him left him feeling disconnected from them.

Many parents feel that they know their children inside out. And, in many ways, this may be true. But our understanding of the nature of our children is always coloured by our own nature. If, for instance, a parent has an Earth constitutional imbalance, they may feel sure their child needs more motherly love when she is struggling, because that is what the parent would want in that situation. In fact, her child, who has a Metal constitutional imbalance, might be most helped by being allowed more space and time on her own.

The way we have been parented and the hopes, dreams and fears we have concerning our children also distort our understanding of them. This means we inevitably project on to them what is not really theirs. Withdrawing our projections involves a degree of self-insight, time, patience and a lot of deep breaths. However, it is one of the most impactful things we can do to improve our connections and therefore be a positive influence as we strive to prevent and heal the mental/emotional difficulties our children have. Living with 'not knowing' is difficult but, combined with being endlessly curious about children, it is often a more helpful stance for the child than assuming we do know.

Looking under the surface

I have heard many parents say that they just do not understand why their child is struggling mentally or emotionally. They may say that she has lived a charmed life, without any trauma, with a loving, stable family, good friends, robust physical health and a happy school life. Their child's struggles may, of course, be due to the child's nature. She may have a very strong proclivity for worry, for example. She may be extremely sensitive and someone who would always have found life challenging.

However, another possible explanation is that the child is responding emotionally to what lies beneath the picture of perfection that her life seems to be. The family may seemingly work as a system, but behind the exterior manifestation are there high levels of strain to keep it all together? The family members may appear to be harmonious but do they actually feel lonely and disconnected from one another? The child may have found a way of enjoying school, but in order to do that has she had to compromise her authenticity? The parents may appear to have a stable marriage, but are they playing a role instead of really communicating?

It is very often what is unspoken and unseen that has the biggest impact on a child. Finding out what that is involves difficult conversations, ruthless honesty and a lot of courage, which may be painful for everybody involved. However, sometimes it is only going through this painful process (often with some kind of professional support) that ultimately helps a child to thrive.

Knowing your limits

There will be times when the right course of action for both parents and practitioners will be to acknowledge that it is beyond their competence to be able to help a particular child sufficiently. For parents, this may mean finding a psychotherapist, psychologist, psychiatrist or acupuncturist who can help support their child. For practitioners of Chinese medicine, it may mean referring the child to a psychotherapist or psychologist either as well as, or instead of, the treatment they are giving.

The art of nurturing the young

The great Sun Simiao wrote that 'there is no *dao* [meaning "skill" or "practice"] among the common people that is greater than the *dao* of nurturing the young'.[2] Nurturing a child, whether as a parent or practitioner, is an art. It takes practice, focus and commitment. It is a skill that needs to be cultivated. It inevitably involves times of not knowing, times when we feel blocked, hopeless or inadequate. During these times, we need to apply the same gentle and forgiving approach to ourselves as we do to the children in our care.

It is important that children and teenagers eat well, take exercise that is appropriate for them, sleep lots and generally follow the lifestyle guidance outlined earlier in this book. But in order to give a child the nurture she needs, our focus needs to be primarily on understanding who she is.

The greatest strength of the Chinese medicine approach is that it allows for this individualised perspective. As the physician Xu Dachun wrote, 'Illnesses may be identical, but the persons suffering from them are different.'[3] It is when we truly hold respect and treat each child as a unique individual that we have the best chance of supporting them to thrive mentally and emotionally. As parents or practitioners this is surely the finest gift we can give them.

Endnotes

1   H. Macpherson and T. Kaptchuk (eds) (1997) *Acupuncture in Practice: Case History Insights from the West* (Edinburgh: Churchill Livingstone), p. xx.

2   S. Wilms (trans.) (2015) *Venerating the Root: Part 2*. Sun Simiao's *Bei Ji Qian Jin Yao Fang*, Volume 5: Paediatrics (Corbett, OR: Happy Goat Productions), p. xviii.

3   P. Unschuld (1990) *Forgotten Traditions of Ancient Chinese Medicine* (Brookline, MA: Paradigm Publications), p. 17.

Appendix 1

Paediatric *Tui Na*

Massage is a wonderful way of calming anxious thoughts and feelings. Massages that target acupuncture channels and points are especially effective. The massage techniques in this appendix are from a Chinese medical system specifically for children, called paediatric *tui na* (*xiao er tui na*). Although traditionally they were used on young children, in my clinic I have found them to be also effective on teenagers.

Before using these massages on a child, there are some general principles of which you need to be aware:

- Unlike many other massage techniques, paediatric *tui na* gains its effectiveness through repetition rather than force.

- Each move is done repetitively for between one and two minutes, depending on the age and nature of the child.

- The moves should be done quite rapidly, although there is no 'set' speed, and to some degree you can use your intuition as to what feels like the right speed for that child. As a very rough guide, you might do approximately two moves per second.

- It's important to massage using a consistent rhythm.

- You should make firm contact with the child, i.e. more than a tickle, but do not need to use any degree of force beyond that.

- Be guided by the child – some children will be more comfortable with firmer pressure; others will be more comfortable with lighter pressure.

- The moves should be done in a sequence, i.e. one after another. Their effect is cumulative, so it will not work to do one move and then another one later in the day.

Massages to calm the *shen*

Paediatric *tui na* contains hundreds of different moves that are effective in the treatment of a wide range of different conditions. The ones below are a selection of moves that all have the action of calming the *shen*. Therefore they can be used on all children experiencing any sort of agitation, restlessness or inability to sleep. It does not matter which particular Element type or what patterns of imbalance the child has.

This sequence of massage should ideally be done once a day, just before bedtime. Additionally, it can also be done at any point during the day if the child is feeling particularly anxious, or before an event that you know may cause the child's anxiety to spike.

> ● **CONTRAINDICATIONS**
>
> Do not massage over cuts, open wounds, severe eczema, cysts or tumours. These massages are aimed at calming a child. If, for whatever reason, a child appears to not enjoy them, or she finds them uncomfortable, then do not persist with them.

Heaven Gate *tianmen*

Location: This is a line on the forehead, which runs from the point between the eyebrows, up the midline of the forehead to the anterior hairline.

Technique: With the pad of the thumb, stroke in a straight line repeatedly upwards from the point between the eyebrows to the anterior hairline.

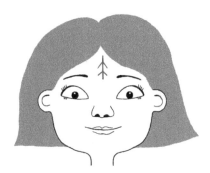

Figure A1.1 Heaven Gate

Water Palace *kangong*

Location: This is a line on the forehead, approximately midway between the tops of the eyebrows and the anterior hairline.

Technique: Starting in the middle of the forehead and using the sides of the pads of both thumbs, repeatedly push outwards with either thumb towards the edges of the forehead.

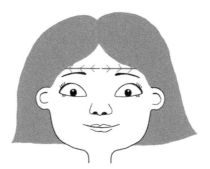

Figure A1.2 Water Palace

Heart Gate *xinmen*

Location: This is a line that runs from the midpoint of the anterior hairline, backwards along the midline at the top of the head, approximately the same distance back as the height of the forehead.

Technique: Starting at the midpoint of the anterior hairline and using the pad of the thumb, repeatedly stroke in a straight line towards the back of the head.

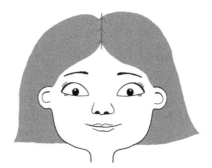

Figure A1.3 Heart Gate

Palace of Toil *laogong*

Location: This is a point that is almost in the centre of the palm of the hand, but slightly towards the thumb side. It is between the second and third meta-carpal bones, which are the bones on the palm that are in line with the index and middle fingers.

Technique: With the pad of your thumb, knead this point for 1–2 minutes. It does not matter in which direction you knead.

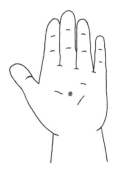

Figure A1.4 Palace of Toil

Small Heavenly Heart *xiaotianxin*

Location: This is a point at the base of the palm of the hand, between the two fleshy areas (the thenar and hypothenar eminences). It is just to the hand side of the wrist crease, i.e. on the hand rather than the arm.

Technique: with the pad of your thumb, knead this point for 1–2 minutes. It does not matter in which direction you knead.

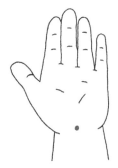

Figure A1.5 Small Heavenly Heart

Milky Way *tianheshui*

Location: This is a line that runs along the middle of the ventral (inner) surface of the forearm, from the wrist crease to the elbow.

Technique: With the pads of two fingers, stroke in a straight line repeatedly from the wrist to the elbow crease.

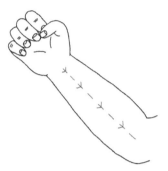

Figure A1.6 Milky Way

Bubbling Spring *yongquan*

Location: This is a point on the sole of the foot. It is between the second and third metatarsal bones, which are the bones that run directly below the second and third toes. It is approximately one-third of the distance between the base of the second toe and the heel.

Technique: With the pad of the thumb, knead this point for 1–2 minutes. It does not matter in which direction you knead.

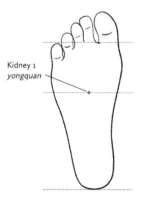

Kidney 1
yongquan

Figure A1.7 Bubbling Spring

Head, Neck and Face Massages

In Chapter 7, we discussed a pattern of imbalance that is common in children who are depressed, called *qi* stagnation. We also mentioned that *qi* stagnation can, in particular, affect the head. These massages are effective at moving or unblocking stuck *qi* in the head and the face. When done consistently over a period of weeks or months, they can positively impact a child's mental/emotional well-being. They also have a very relaxing short-term effect.

Head massage

These massages are done along acupuncture channels which run over the head. The easiest way to do them is to ask the child to lie down, and to stand behind the top of her head.

● **CONTRAINDICATION**
Never perform the head massages on a baby younger than two years old. This is the age by which the fontanelle (soft spots) on the head will have closed up.

Method

- Using the pads of the thumbs, massage with some force along the channels as shown in Figure A2.1.

- Always massage from the front of the head backwards towards the top of the head.

- Make small circular movements with your thumbs as you massage along the line.

- Check in with the child as you do it and adjust the pressure you are using accordingly.

- Depending on the age and maturity of the child, you can do these massages for anywhere between five and fifteen minutes, once a day. Just before bedtime is a particularly good time for them, because of their ability to promote relaxation.

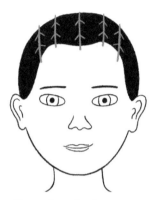

Figure A2.1 Head massage

Neck massage

The neck massage described here is as powerful as it is simple. From a Chinese medicine perspective, it helps to descend *qi* and promotes the smooth flow of *qi* in several key acupuncture channels. From a Western perspective, it helps to regulate the vagus nerve, the smooth functioning of which is understood to be important in the management of anxiety.

Method

1. With the pads of three fingers, simply stroke downwards as shown in Figure A2.2.

2. Repeat this action with a steady rhythm and a pressure that is acceptable to the child.

3. Continue for approximately one minute on each side of the neck.

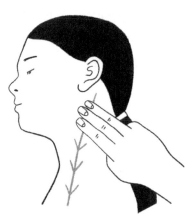

Figure A2.2 Calming neck massage

Face massage

These massages are done along acupuncture channels and points on the face. Sometimes they follow exactly the lines of an acupuncture channel, and sometimes they move between acupuncture points on various different channels. They help to enliven the senses of the child, thereby easing the symptoms of depression. Like the head massages, they are also effective at promoting relaxation through their ability to move blocked *qi*. Depending on the age and maturity of the child, you can do these massages for anywhere between five and fifteen minutes, once a day. Just before bedtime is a particularly good time for them, because of their ability to promote relaxation.

These face massages must be done with much lighter pressure than the head massages.

Method

1. Massage the acupuncture point *yintang*, which is in the middle of the eyebrows.

2. With the sides of your thumbs, stroke across the forehead from the midline outwards.

3. Massage the acupuncture point *taiyang*, which is on the temple, in the depression lateral to and slightly below the outer point of the eyebrow.

4. Place a thumb either side of the base of the nose. Massage outwards across the cheek bone with both thumbs until you reach the front of the ear.

5. Place your thumbs and index finger in the midpoint of the chin, your thumb below the chin and your index finger above it. Massage outwards along the jaw bone, until you reach the end of it, which is just below the ear.

Figure A2.3 illustrates the sequence of face massages just described.

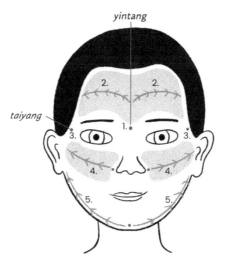

Figure A2.3 Face massage

Appendix 3

Auriculotherapy

Auriculotherapy is often used by acupuncturists, in conjunction with, or instead of, body acupuncture. The ear is a microsystem of the entire body. There are several acupuncture points on the ear which help to soothe the nervous system and calm anxiety.

The easiest and most effective way to stimulate the points at home is by sticking tiny vaccaria seeds onto the relevant point. The seeds (which are stuck to a piece of self-adhesive tape) are readily available to buy online (just search for 'vaccaria ear seeds'). They work away in the background while the child is able to get on with her life.

● **CONTRAINDICATION**
Do not use ear seeds on babies or children under the age of three.

Method

1. Ear points are usually tender – to help locate the point, probe the area using a fine object, such as a toothpick, to find the most tender place in the vicinity of the point.

2. Apply the sticker to the ear and press it firmly in place.

3. Only apply the sticker to one ear at a time.

4. After two to three days, remove the sticker.

5. If necessary, apply a fresh sticker to the opposite ear.

Figure A3.1 shows two points most commonly used in the treatment of anxiety in children, namely *shenmen* and Spleen. One option is to put stickers on both points. However, if you would prefer to keep it simple, just using the point *shenmen* alone can have a beneficial impact.

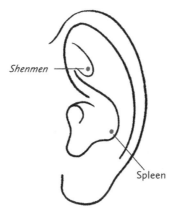

Figure A3.1 Auricular points for anxiety

Appendix 4

Dissipating Stuck Emotions

It can take some time to get to the root of a child's distress and for the child to make the necessary changes to their life. In the meantime, there are some effective tools that can be used that help to dissipate stuck emotions. For instance, you might be caring for a child whose tendency is to have several outbursts of anger a day, or to be beset by worry every bedtime. The suggestions contained here are to help you and a child for whom you care in the short term, while the more long-term changes can begin to be made.

Helping a child who is stuck in a lack of joy or sadness

- Create opportunities for laughter every day: for instance, watch something funny or play a funny game.

- Work on intimacy: create opportunities for the child to spend time with those she feels loved by and close to.

- Create activities that spark joy in the child and that light her inner fire.

- Place a vaccaria seed (see Appendix 3) on the ear acupuncture point *shenmen* (Figure A3.1).

Helping a child who is stuck in worry

- Get moving: there comes a time when it is no longer helpful to keep talking things over. The child needs to get moving (nothing vigorous, just gentle movement is fine) to encourage her *qi* out of her head and to free it up.

- Do something practical: create something, for example, bake cookies or do some kind of craft activity.

- Turn thought into action: if the worries are focused on something that needs to be done, setting about that thing is often the most effective way of easing the worries.

- Place a vaccaria seed (see Appendix 3) on the ear acupuncture point Spleen (Figure A3.1).

Helping a child who is stuck in fear

- Take all unnecessary pressures off the child (e.g. the requirement to do music practice, household chores, etc.).

- Create an environment of safety, where the adults are calm and present and life is as predictable as possible.

- Reduce stimulation levels as much as possible.

- Place a vaccaria seed on the acupuncture point Kidney 1 *yongquan* (see Figure A1.7).

Helping a child who is stuck in anger

- Encourage exercise which, depending on the child, can be quite vigorous: this helps to make *qi* flow.

- Support an older child to find a safe way to bring the anger up and out, e.g. beating a pillow against a bed.

- Find a creative outlet: the counterpart to anger is creativity.

- Stream-of-consciousness writing. This idea is borrowed from *The Artist's Way* by Julia Cameron, and I have adapted it for children.[1] It involves sitting down for five minutes and continually writing. The only rule is that you cannot pause writing. It does not matter what comes out (it might be complete nonsense), and nobody is going to see it. After a few minutes, this activity bypasses the conscious mind and the emotions that were stored in the unconscious begin to surface and be revealed in the writing. Throw the paper away afterwards. It should be done daily.

- Place a vaccaria seed on the acupuncture point Liver 3 *taichong* (see Figure A4.1).

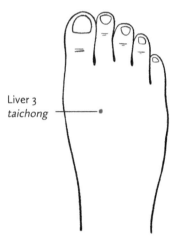

Liver 3
taichong

Figure A4.1 Acupuncture point Liver 3 taichong

Endnote

1   J. Cameron (1995) *The Artist's Way: A Spiritual Path to Higher Creativity* (London: Pan Books).

Appendix 5

Finding a Paediatric Acupuncturist

Acupuncture is a wonderful tool to help children maintain and recover their mental/emotional well-being. Because their *qi* is *yang* in nature, children respond readily to minimal intervention. What's more, acupuncture can be delivered without the use of needles. There are many other modalities – including low-level laser and different types of medical massage to name but two – that can be used instead. Having said that, most children are quite happy to be treated with needles, which are so fine that they can barely be felt, and which are inserted and then immediately withdrawn.

It is important that you choose an acupuncturist for your child who has postgraduate training in paediatrics, although most well-trained acupuncturists will be competent to treat teenagers.

You can find a database of paediatric acupuncture specialists, as well as more information about paediatric acupuncture, at the Hub of Paediatric Acupuncture website: www.paediatricacupuncture.co.uk.

Bibliography

Avern, R. (2019) *Acupuncture for Babies, Children and Teenagers: Treating Both the Illness and the Child*. London: Singing Dragon.

Blyth, D. and Lampert, G. (2015) *Chinese Dietary Wisdom*. Reading: Nutshell Press.

Cameron, J. (1995) *The Artist's Way: A Spiritual Path to Higher Creativity*. London: Pan Books.

Chatterjee, R. (2018) *The 4 Pillar Plan*. London: Penguin Life.

Chatterjee, R. (2018) *The Stress Solution*. London: Penguin Life.

Cowan, S. (2012) *Fire Child, Water Child*. Oakland, CA: New Harbinger.

Damour, L. (2019) *Under Pressure: Confronting the Epidemic of Stress and Anxiety in Girls*. New York: Ballantine Books.

Deadman, P. (2016) *Live Well, Live Long*. Hove: JCM Publications.

Dechar, L. (2006) *Five Spirits*. New York: Lantern Books.

Flaws, B. (2006) *A Handbook of TCM Paediatrics*. Boulder, CO: Blue Poppy Press.

Hari, J. (2019) *Lost Connections: Why You're Depressed and How to Find Hope*. London: Bloomsbury.

Hicks, A. and Hicks, J. (1999) *Healing Your Emotions*. London: Thorsons.

Hicks, A., Hicks, J. and Mole, P. (2011) *Five Element Constitutional Acupuncture*. Edinburgh: Churchill Livingstone.

Hohnen, B., Gilmour, J. and Murphy, T. (2020) *The Incredible Teenage Brain: Everything You Need to Know to Unlock Your Teen's Potential*. London: Jessica Kingsley Publishers.

Kaptchuk, T. (1983) *Chinese Medicine: The Web that Has No Weaver*. London: Random House.

Larre, C. and Rochat de la Vallée, E. (1996) *The Seven Emotions*. Cambridge: Monkey Press.

Maciocia, G. (2005) *The Foundations of Chinese Medicine*. Edinburgh: Churchill Livingstone.

Maciocia, G. (2009) *The Psyche in Chinese Medicine*. London: Churchill Livingstone.

Mole, P. (2007) *Acupuncture for Body, Mind and Spirit*. Oxford: How To Books.

Montakab, H. (2012) *Acupuncture for Insomnia: Sleep and Dreams in Chinese Medicine*. Stuttgart: Thieme.

Nestor, J. (2020) *Breath: The New Science of a Lost Art*. London: Penguin Life.

Perry, P. (2019) *The Book You Wish Your Parents Had Read*. London: Penguin Life.

Rosen, R. (2018) *Heart Shock*. London: Singing Dragon.

Rossi, E. (2007) *Shen: Psycho-Emotional Aspects of Chinese Medicine*. London: Churchill Livingstone.

Rossi, E. (2011) *Paediatrics in Chinese Medicine*. Barnet: Donica.

Samuel, J. (2020) *This Too Shall Pass: Stories of Change, Crisis and Hopeful Beginnings*. London: Penguin Life.

Scott, J. and Barlow, T. (1999) *Acupuncture in the Treatment of Children*. Seattle, WA: Eastland Press.

Sterman, A. (2020) *Welcoming Food Book 1: Energetics of Food and Healing*. New York: Classical Wellness Press.

Stossel, S. (2014) *My Age of Anxiety*. London: Windmill Books.

Vohra, S. (2018) *Mental Health in Children and Young People*. London: Sheldon Press.

Wilms, S. (trans.) (2013) *Venerating the Root: Part 1*. Sun Simiao's *Bei Ji Qian Jin Yao Fang*, Volume 5: Paediatrics. Corbett, OR: Happy Goat Productions.

Wilms, S. (trans.) (2015) *Venerating the Root: Part 2*. Sun Simiao's *Bei Ji Qian Jin Yao Fang*, Volume 5: Paediatrics. Corbett, OR: Happy Goat Productions.

Yousheng, L. (2014) *Let the Radiant Yang Shine Forth: Lectures on Virtue*, translated by L. Zuozhi and S. Wilms. Corbett, OR: Happy Goat Productions.

Index

Note: Illustrations are indicated by page numbers in *italics*